# THE HE
# HANDBOOK

## A Special Edition for Our Patients at North Ridge Medical Center and Heart Institute

**A**S **YOU** check into the hospital for heart surgery, you are embarking on one of the most serious and critical experiences of your life. This handbook, provided by your surgeons, will give you some insight into what your heart operation will mean—in terms of both risks and benefits—and also help you and your family survive the emotional strain of surgery and recovery. You'll find the book thorough and easy-to-use, with an exhaustive index, diagrams, and full glossary of medical terms. A list of additional resources is also provided.

Communication and information are vital to coping successfully with any medical problem. In today's world of instant communications—with so much medical knowledge being disbursed on television and in other media—many people have a *little* medical knowledge that can be dangerous. It can lead them to false conclusions about a problem they or their family may have. Thus, as you or a family member goes through the experience of heart surgery, never hesitate to ask questions of the many professionals you will encounter along the way. And if they don't take the time to answer, it may be time to get a second opinion about your care. As you'll read in Chapter One of this handbook, patients who are counseled before and after surgery—who receive complete, accurate information on what to expect every step of the way—recover more successfully than patients who do not. That's why we've written this book and provided you this copy. We trust you'll find it a helpful guide and companion.

## A Brief Anatomy Lesson

As our diagrams in Appendix II show, the heart is a hollow muscle containing four chambers. Blood enters at one end and exits at the other. Venous blood—dark and depleted of oxygen after its trip through the body—enters the heart by way of the cavae (tubes the size of your thumb) to collect in the first upper chamber, the right atrium. From here it is pumped under low pressure through the tricuspid valve—so called for its three parts—into the right ventricle below. This thin-walled, muscular chamber squeezes the blood through the pulmonary valve into the pulmonary artery, another large, thumb-sized tube. Through this artery the blood passes to the lungs, where it picks up oxygen and gives up carbon dioxide, turning a bright red.

The freshly oxygenated blood then flows into another chamber of the heart called the left atrium, also a low pressure area. This chamber pumps the blood into the left ventricle below through the mitral valve (named for its resemblance to a bishop's miter, with the two halves suspended by strands like a parachute). The left ventricle is the main pumping chamber of the heart. Being a large and thick-muscled compartment, it creates the pressure necessary to pump the blood throughout the body, by way of the aortic valve through the aorta. The aorta is a large, hose-sized artery, with many branches leading to all the organs of the body. The first few of these branches lead to the heart itself and are called the coronary arteries.

## Types of Heart Surgery

Most heart surgery today is performed to remedy blockages in the coronary arteries, known as *bypass surgery*. In fact, this type of surgery gave rise to this book, and we describe it in detail later on. Briefly, when the coronary arteries are blocked, a heart attack may occur, causing part of the heart muscle to die. If the blocked artery is large, the muscle still living may be insufficient to sustain the heart's pumping action and the patient may die. In life-threatening situations, heart surgery is necessary to construct a detour—a bypass—for blood to flow freely to the heart muscle. This is done by using the saphenous veins from the leg or the internal mammary arteries near the breastbone, grafting them from the aorta to the threatened muscle.

Atherosclerosis, the disease that causes the arteries to become blocked, is an ongoing process that bypass surgery cannot stop. Thus the grafts used for bypass can also harden and develop blockage, particularly the veins. Ten years after surgery, about half the vein grafts are still functioning while close to ninety-two percent of the artery grafts are still functioning at that time. Unfortunately, the arteries cannot always be used, because they may not be large enough or long enough to make the detour.

Diseases of the heart valves, on the other hand, are less common today due to the alleviation of such diseases as rheumatic fever, which affects the valves in childhood but does not cause problems until many years later. Sometimes valves simply wear out from use over seven or eight decades. This is especially true of the aortic valve, which is subjected to the greatest strain. Diseases of the heart valves involve *leakage,* allowing blood to flow back through the valve, or *blockage,* which prevents blood from flowing forward. In either case, if the problem is severe enough, the valve may have to be repaired. More commonly, it is replaced, either with a tissue valve such as the specially modified and treated pig valve—the "porcine xenograft"—or with a mechanical valve of metal or plastic. Which type of valve we use will depend on your age and other factors.

Heart valve surgery is true open-heart surgery. In coronary bypass operations, we work only on the surface of the heart. In valve surgery, we work within its chambers.

## Heart Surgery Associates

Heart Surgery Associates is a group of board-certified heart and lung surgeons who devoted their training and now devote their practice to heart, blood-vessel, and lung surgery. Our five members together offer almost 100 years of training and practical experience. Our office is located at 5601 North Dixie Highway, Suite 214, in Oakland Park, Florida (305-942-7083). Adjacent to and connected with the North Ridge Medical Center, this location allows us immediate access to our patients in the hospital. Please read about our staff following this introduction.

## Finances

The cost of heart surgery is of great concern to many patients and their families. The care and recovery of our patients is of primary concern to us, and while important, payment is secondary. Our staff will be most happy to discuss the financial aspects of surgery with the patient and family; we do not want your concerns to deter you from seeking proper medical care.

Heart Surgery Associates is associated with quality Health Maintenance Organizations (HMOs), and our fee schedule is accepted by insurance carriers.

## A Final Note

Education is the most important factor in going through heart surgery with the least mental trauma. Again, it is to that end we have provided you this book. While we're certain it will answer many of your questions, rest assured that the lines of communication with the staff at North Ridge and Heart Surgery Associates are always open.

**Heart Surgery Associates**
Fort Lauderdale, Florida

# Heart Surgery Associates

**James R. Jude, M. D., F. A. C. S.** (Fellow of the American College of Surgeons), was born in Minnesota. He received his college education at the College of St. Thomas in St. Paul, Minnesota, and was graduated from the University of Minnesota Medical School in 1953. He interned at the Johns Hopkins Hospital in Baltimore, Maryland, where he remained for his residency in General and Thoracic and Cardiovascular Surgery for the following eight years, with two years of service at the National Institutes of Health in Bethesda.

While at Johns Hopkins, he developed Cardiopulmonary Resuscitation (CPR) with Drs. William Kouwenhoven and G. Guy Knickerbocker. In 1964, he came to South Florida to the University of Miami School of Medicine as Professor of Surgery and as Chief of Thoracic and Cardiovascular Surgery at Jackson Memorial Hospital. In 1971, he entered the private practice of Heart, Lung, and Blood Vessel Surgery.

Dr. Jude is certified by the American Board of Surgery (1962) and the American Board of Thoracic and Cardiovascular Surgery (1962). He is a Fellow of the American College of Chest Physicians and the American College of Cardiology. He is a member of the American Surgical Association, the Southern Surgical Association, the Southern Thoracic Surgery Association, the American Association for Thoracic Surgery, the Society of Thoracic Surgery, the Society for Vascular Surgery, the Society of University Surgeons, and the International Surgery Association.

He is also a member of the Dade County and Florida Medical Associations, the American Lung Association, the American Heart Association, and the Florida Thoracic Society. In addition to having published many scientific articles, he is the co-author of two books, *Cardiopulmonary Resuscitation* and this handbook.

**Robert Cline, M. D., F. A. C. S.,** was born in Iowa. He was educated at Duke University in Durham, North Carolina, graduating from its School of Medicine in 1963. He interned at the New York Hospital and took his residency in General Surgery and Thoracic and Cardiovascular Surgery at the Duke University Medical Center from 1964 to 1971.

Dr. Cline is certified by the American Board of Surgery (1971) and the American Board of Thoracic Surgery (1971). He is a Fellow of the American College of Cardiology and a member of the Society of Thoracic Surgeons, the Southern Thoracic Surgery Association, the Society of Air Force Clinical Surgeons, and the International Cardiovascular Society. He is also a member of the Broward County Medical Society, the Florida Medical Association, and the American Heart Association.

Dr. Cline has been on the staff of North Ridge Hospital since 1976 and founded the Second Chance Heart Club. He has been associated with Dr. Jude in Heart Surgery Associates since 1978.

**Hugh Dennis, M. D., F. A. C. S.,** was born in South Carolina. He received his undergraduate education at Davidson College in North Carolina and his medical degree from Tulane University School of Medicine in 1975. His internship was at Charity Hospital in New Orleans, and his General Surgical Residency at Tulane University and Charity Hospital. His residency in Thoracic and Cardiovascular Surgery was at the St. Louis University Hospitals in 1982. Following that, he joined Drs. Jude and Cline in Heart Surgery Associates.

Dr. Dennis is certified by the American Board of Surgery (1980) and the American Board of Thoracic Surgery (1983). He is a member of the Society of Thoracic Surgeons, the Southern Thoracic Surgery Association, and the Florida Society of Thoracic and Cardiovascular Surgeons. He is also a member of the Broward Medical Association and the Florida and American Medical Associations.

**Stuart Boe, M. D., F. A. C. S.,** was born in Oregon. His undergraduate education was at Brown University in Providence, Rhode Island, where he also received his medical degree in 1975 and a Master's in Medical Science in 1978. He interned at Rhode Island Hospital in 1976, receiving his training in General Surgery. His residency in Thoracic and Cardiovascular Surgery was at the Allegheny General Hospital in Pittsburgh, Pennsylvania, and the Deborah Heart and Lung Center in Browns Mills, New Jersey.

Dr. Boe is certified by the American Board of Surgery (1983) and the American Board of Thoracic Surgery (1985). He is a Fellow of the American College of Cardiology. He is a member of the New York Academy of Science and the American Association for the Advancement of Science.

Dr. Boe came to South Florida in 1983 and became associated with Heart Surgery Associates in 1987.

**Frank Catinella, M. D.,** was born in New York City. His undergraduate studies were at Notre Dame University, and he obtained his medical degree from the New York University School of Medicine in 1978.

Dr. Catinella interned at the North Shore University Hospital in New York and received his training in General Surgery at New York University Medical Center and at Maimonides Medical Center in New York. His residency in Thoracic and Cardiovascular Surgery was at Rush-Presbyterian-St. Luke's Medical Center in Chicago, Illinois.

Dr. Catinella is certified by the American Board of Surgery (1986) and is board-eligible for certification by the American Board of Thoracic Surgery. He is a Fellow of the American College of Chest Physicians and a member of the Association for Academic Surgery and the American Medical Association. He joined Heart Surgery Associates in 1988.

**THE PHYSICIANS ASSISTANTS** of Heart Surgery Associates have had training similar to two years of medical school. **Stuart Nesbitt** was trained at Emory University in Atlanta, Georgia. **Richard Monti** received his Physicians Assistant training at the University of Nebraska Medical Center in Omaha. **David Stahler** received his certification from Alderson-Broaddus College in Philippi, West Virginia. **Charles Gery**'s Allied Health certificate as a Physicians Assistant was awarded by the University of Alabama in Birmingham. **Edward Zapor** received his Surgeon's Assistant training at the University of Alabama in Birmingham. All are certified by the National Commission on Certification of Physician Assistants.

# THE HEART SURGERY HANDBOOK

# THE HEART SURGERY HANDBOOK

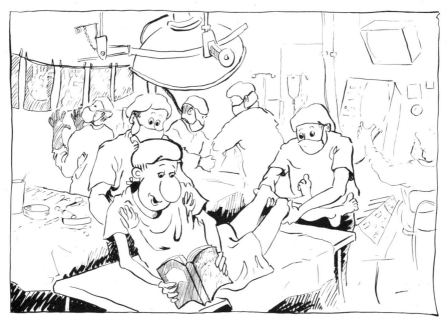

# A PATIENT'S GUIDE

**Carol Cohan M.A.**
**June B. Pimm Ph.D.**
**James R. Jude M.D.**

The Pickering Press

The Pickering Press
2665 South Bayshore Drive, Suite 601, Miami, FL 33133

Library of Congress Cataloging-in-Publication Data

Cohan, Carol, 1943-
  The heart surgery handbook.

  Bibliography: p.
  Includes index.
  1. Aortocoronary bypass—Popular works. 2. Aortocoronary bypass—Psychological aspects. 3. Depression, Mental—Prevention. 4. Patient education. I. Pimm, June B., 1927-   . II. Jude, James R. III. Title.
  RD598.C52      1988      617'.412      88-9827
  ISBN 0-949485-11-2
  ISBN 0-940495-08-2  (pbk.)
  Illustrations by Astrid Weinkle

# ABOUT THE AUTHORS

**Carol Cohan M.A.** has written for several of the National Institutes of Health, as well as for medical schools, hospitals, rehabilitation centers, and ambulatory care facilities. Her articles on a wide range of medical subjects have been published in close to a dozen specialty publications. In 1986 her work on magnetic resonance imaging received the Florida Medical Association's Award for Excellence in Medical Journalism. For ten years, she was a member of the writing faculty at the American University. In that capacity, she taught business writing to members of the White House staff and in 1980 won the University's Outstanding Teaching award. Ms. Cohan is a graduate of the University of Maryland and Columbia University.

**June B. Pimm Ph.D.** has been a clinical psychologist in private practice for thirty years. She has conducted research and published widely in the area of developmental psychology and behavioral medicine. In 1970 she wrote and directed the award winning film "Child Behavior Equals You" and in 1984 co-authored the book *Psychological Risks of Coronary Bypass Surgery* (Plenum Press). A graduate of McGill University, Dr. Pimm has taught at Carleton University and the University of Miami Medical School.

**James R. Jude M.D.** Cardiovascular Surgeon in the private practice of heart surgery, graduated from the University of Minnesota School of Medicine in 1953. He received his surgical training at Johns Hopkins under the renowned surgeon, Dr. Alfred Blalock. At Johns Hopkins, together with Dr. William Kouwenhoven and Dr. Guy Knickerbocker, he developed cardiopulmonary resuscitation (CPR). For this work he received the Award of Merit of the American Heart Association. Subsequently, he was Chief of Heart and Lung Surgery at the University of Miami School of Medicine, where he remains Clinical Professor of Surgery. Currently he is Chief of Cardiovascular and Thoracic Surgery at the North Ridge Heart Institute in Fort Lauderdale, Florida, and a Thoracic and Cardiovascular Surgeon at Mercy Hospital in Miami, Florida.

# ACKNOWLEDGMENTS

This book would not have been possible without the support of the American Heart Association, Miami Chapter, which provided funds for our research on depression and coronary bypass surgery.

Abundant thanks go to the physicians who generously participated in this project: Drs. Richard P. Cohen, Paul DeWitt, Malcolm Dorman, Thomas Gentsch, Charles Hyams, Parry B. Larson, Susan Light, John Lister, Norton Luger, James Margolis, Jerry Stolzenberg, Ernest Traad, and Jonathan Tuerk. We are also grateful to Jeff Raines, Ph.D.; Andrea Fisch, R.N.; Shirley Haskell and Memorial Hospital's chapter of Mended Hearts; Sally Kolitz, Ph.D.; Patti Perlman, Psy.D.; Paul Stickney; and Judith Wolfe, M.S.W. Thanks, too, to the scores of patients who shared their confidences so that future patients and their families might benefit. Our deepest gratitude goes to Catherine Tuerk, M.A., R.N., C.S., a wise and sensitive psychotherapist.

Much of the research for this book took place at North Ridge Medical Center/Heart Institute and never could have been accomplished without the enthusiastic assistance of the fine, caring professional staff. Most of all, thank you to Barbara Friedman, R.N., M.S. In addition, we also thank Karen Baumann, P.A.-C.; Carol Dwyer, R.N., M.S.N.; Ali Ghahramani, M.D.; Sue Jones, R.P.T.; Richard Monti, P.A.-C.; Stuart Nesbitt, P.A.-C.; Cindy Porter, R.N.; David Stahler, P.A.-C.; Alan Stillerman, R.T.; and Margo Snedden.

We are indebted to Bess Marder and Robert Pimm for their editorial talents. Thanks also to Bernice Johnson, Raymond Marat, and Joseph R. Feist, Ph.D., for their contributions to this manuscript. Finally, we appreciate the efforts and commitment of Charity Johnson, Manager/Editor at The Pickering Press, and Michele Jean, who typed the manuscript.

# TABLE OF CONTENTS

x

# FOREWORD

As a practicing cardiologist over the past twenty-five years, I have been struck by the number of patients, friends and acquaintances who have complained to me of how inadequately they were prepared to meet the psychological stress of heart surgery.

In today's world of multispecialty team medicine, failure of communication is an increasing problem, and while many patients are satisfied with a photocopied instruction sheet and a hasty viewing of a video film, many of the others are expecting a deeper and more thorough understanding of their apprehension and a fuller explanation of the strange new world that they are about to encounter.

*The Heart Surgery Handbook* is the answer to their prayers (and mine). In this book, the authors take the prospective patient step by step through the surgical process from diagnosis to the resumption of activities and a return to the workplace. Their years of experience in researching hundreds of patients undergoing cardiac surgery place them in a unique position to provide the most appropriate information, advice and encouragement to candidates for heart surgery. Chapter by chapter, the prospective patient is led through the events he will experience in the most knowledgeable and reassuring manner. The purpose of this book is to minimize the risk of anxiety, frustration and depression during the period surrounding the operation which is so often the cause of delayed recovery, increased risk of complications and reduced surgical benefit.

For the discerning patient about to undergo heart surgery, as well as his loved ones, this book will be like a trusted companion and knowledgeable advisor and, in my opinion, it should never be far from the bedside.

Dr. R. F. P. Cronin,
FRCP (London), FRCP (Canada)
Former Director, Canadian Heart Association
Former Dean, Faculty of Medicine, McGill University

# INTRODUCTION

## The Problem

Thousands of people have been disappointed with the results of their coronary artery bypass graft surgery. Although their surgery was successful, they do not feel a sense of strength and vigor. Some are oppressed by depression. Others feel physical malaise. Still others find that the pieces of their lives lie as disconnected as an unsolved jigsaw puzzle.

Not long ago, the problem was illustrated poignantly by a middle-aged couple on the golf course. The husband, appearing strong and muscular, played his first shot with the skill of an experienced athlete. However, as he prepared to hit his second shot, his wife turned to a friend and said fearfully, "I hope he plays well. He's just recovered from bypass surgery and is still so depressed; I feel inadequate to help him."

## The Study

Because this problem afflicts so many people, we devised a study to help us understand it and solve it. We hypothesized that most patients who failed to feel well despite successful surgery were suffering from depression and that, if we could relieve their depression, they would recover more quickly and fully.

What followed was the Miami Heart Institute Study, a three-year project which assessed depression in bypass patients and evaluated the effectiveness of specific short-term supportive counseling in alleviating it. The study, which ran at the Miami Heart Institute and South Miami Hospital, confirmed our suspicions. As several dozen other studies have since verified, we found that heart surgery leaves approximately one-third of patients depressed. Of our patients who received *standard care,* 28% developed such severe depression that it prevented them from feeling their surgery had been successful. These patients remained depressed for up to three years. However, our research also showed that when the psychological adjustment of patients and their families received *special attention,* patients fared better. With supportive counseling, the incidence dropped to 6%. Most important of all, the study showed that patients who were likely to suffer from enduring depression shared certain characteristics, and therefore it was possible to predict which patients needed counseling most.

The counseling which the Miami Heart Institute Study set out to test follows the guidelines for crisis intervention devised by Gerald Caplan, M.D., Director of Harvard University Medical School's Laboratory of Community Psychiatry. Many psychologists turn to crisis intervention, which is specifically designed to ease the psychological consequences of normal life crises, when they work with communities after earthquakes, violence of various kinds, and other tragedies. Since heart surgery has many characteristics in common with other life crises, we conjectured that crisis intervention would help patients cope with it.

To test the validity of this theory, we chose 104 patients of similar profile—all were male heads of households whose roles had changed temporarily because of their illness and surgery. We divided them into two groups, assessed their levels of depression before surgery, then followed them for three years to assess medical progress and measure depression. All patients received whatever counseling and support surgical patients normally receive at the two participating hospitals. In addition, patients in one group received crisis intervention counseling from the day before surgery until eight weeks after they were home. Patients in both groups were reevaluated four weeks after counseling ended. Three years after surgery, we succeeded in locating thirty-four of the patients, whom we interviewed and tested again.

Before surgery, patients in both groups took a battery of nine self-administered psychological tests to measure their levels of depression as well as a number of personality dimensions. Several of these tools proved extremely helpful. To measure depression, we used the *Beck Depression Inventory*, which asks patients to endorse or reject statements like "I feel bad or unworthy a good part of the time" and "I feel I am being punished." These items are intended to reveal the extent to which respondents have adopted a pessimistic attitude toward life. The *Beck Depression Inventory* measures the way people think and feel, including physical symptoms, since each of these factors can reflect depression.

Patients also responded to the *Rotter Locus of Control Scale*. This test reveals whether people believe they control their lives or whether they feel their lives are controlled by an outside force. People who, in Rotter's words, have an *internal locus of control* would affirm statements like "for a well-prepared student there is rarely, if ever, an unfair test" or "becoming successful is a matter of hard work; luck has little or nothing to do with it." In contrast, those with an *external locus of control* would probably believe that "without the right breaks, one cannot be an effective leader" or "che sera, sera."

Another valuable measure was an adapted form of the *Recent Life Changes Questionnaire*. This tool, developed by psychiatrists Thomas Holmes and Richard Rahe, lists 100 common life occurrences, each with a point value corresponding to the intensity of its emotional impact. By indicating which events they had experienced within the preceding six months, respondents reveal how much they taxed their coping resources during that period.

We found that 20% of all patients were depressed the day before their operations and all patients experienced intermittent depression during the days and weeks following surgery. But three months after surgery, depression fell to 14% among the counseling group while it rose to 24% among those who received standard care. At the end of three years, an additional 4% of patients in the second group became depressed, while the number of depressed in the counseling group dropped to just 6%. More significantly, twice as many depressed patients died or experienced serious medical complications at both measuring points.

The results of this study were first published in *Psychological Risks of Coronary Bypass Surgery,* by June B. Pimm, Ph.D., and Joseph R. Feist, Ph.D., a book intended for medical and mental health professionals. It was reviewed by *Contemporary Psychology* and described as an "excellent example of a well-designed and controlled research program in a clinical setting." Because of the thoroughness and care with which the study was conducted, it "represents the practice of health psychology at its best."

Interestingly, our results are consistent with those of another project involving short-term counseling for patients with heart disease. In a McGill University study of nearly 500 heart attack patients, individually tailored assistance was offered to reduce stress. In an average of five to six hours of private counseling over a year's time, nurses provided patients with emotional support, referrals to health care professionals, and information about heart disease and medication. This intervention reduced mortality by 50%.

## The Solution

The crisis intervention which our counselors provided consisted largely of giving patients and their families information about surgery and recovery, and helping them solve any accompanying problems. This book is an adaptation of that counseling. It has been written for future patients and their families. In the forthcoming pages, we explore each stage of the heart surgery experience, from the time bypass is recommended until months after surgery is completed. We discuss what other patients encountered at each stage, problems that arose, and solutions that worked for a variety of people with different personalities and coping styles.

Unlike other books on heart surgery, *The Heart Surgery Handbook* does not delve deeply into heart disease and its treatment alternatives. Rather, it is designed specifically as a prescription for coping with them. If you know what to expect, if you can perceive your problems as normal, and if you can identify solutions which seem appropriate for you, the problems become less threatening.

The underlying theory here is not unique to heart surgery. In most of life, knowing what to expect makes the unknown more predictable and therefore more manageable. Applying this theory to other areas of medicine has proven quite profitable. For example, when pregnant women learn about childbirth and practice exercises to help them cope with labor, they often reduce the intensity of their pain and need less medication. An innovative approach to patients recuperating from heart attacks also illustrates this principle. Patients recovered unusually quickly when, in addition to standard patient education, they received a short course in coronary heart disease and its treatment. They responded well to watching their electrocardiogram (EKG) tracings and exercising under supervision.

Similarly, abdominal surgery patients benefited from expanded preoperative instruction. The patients who learned what to expect in the postoperative period, how to relax by deep breathing, and how to move easily left the hospital more than two days earlier and needed less pain medication than patients who received standard patient education. Gynecological surgery patients confirmed the point as well. When they received information designed to quiet preoperative fear, help them manage postoperative pain, and speed recovery, they suffered less anxiety, as measured by lowered blood pressure and heart rate.

Most heart surgery patients, when asked, agree it is important to know exactly what to expect every step of the way. Moreover, their experiences suggest that when they have time to assimilate the information slowly, they process it more effectively and can call upon it more reliably than when they are bombarded with it immediately before surgery. Several patients who had to undergo emergency bypass and were given all their instructions in the minutes before they were put to sleep experienced panic when they woke up, whereas those who had time to prepare had a greater sense of calm and control.

If there is a sweeping conclusion that we can draw from the Miami Heart Institute Study and from the additional research that went into this book, it is that no one goes into or emerges from heart surgery in exactly the same way as anyone else. More important, there is no right or wrong way to approach the procedure or manage recovery. When learning that he should have surgery, one patient headed straight for the golf course. Another went to his safety deposit box to review his will. A third arranged a candlelit dinner with his wife, where they reflected upon the years when their marriage was young and their children were small. By the same token, you may approach this book by turning directly to the chapter on the intensive care unit. Someone else may prefer to begin with the interconnection of mind and body, which is discussed in chapter ten. Some may read from cover to cover, while others may prefer to select only isolated sections. In using this book, as in undergoing surgery, you would do best to follow the course that feels most comfortable and reassuring to you.

Chapter One
# BYPASSING DEPRESSION

"If only I had known what to expect, this
would have been so much easier."
*— common patient complaint*


Just twenty years ago, when Drs. Rene Favaloro and
Dudley Johnson developed coronary artery bypass graft
surgery, the notion of surgically improving blood flow to
the heart seemed a radical experiment. Within fifteen
years, however, more than a million such operations were
performed, and now it is more common than any other
major surgery. Today, there are some 230,000 bypass
operations a year in the United States alone, and for good
reason. For the right patient, bypass surgery promises
more years of active, high-quality life than any other
treatment.

Although the idea of opening the chest and repairing
the heart seems ominous, the surgery has a superb 97%
success rate. Considering that many patients who undergo bypass surgery are seventy-five, eighty, eighty-five
years old and suffering from chronic diseases characteristic of old age, this figure is indeed impressive. Among
younger, otherwise healthy people, the statistics are even
better.

Most patients recover without major incident. Within
hours after surgery, they commonly show healthy color in
their faces even though they are still asleep from anesthesia. Within a few days, most stroll the hospital corridors
chatting with nurses and visitors. In less than two weeks,
even some octogenarians are strong enough to walk outside on warm, windless days.

"My gracious, there goes Molly," one young woman exclaimed as she watched her eighty-four-year-old neighbor carefully but purposefully walk down the block thirteen days after a triple bypass.

This kind of dramatic progress is one factor which makes the surgery so desirable. Ironically, this dramatic speed of recovery may cause problems for some patients.

Inured to a procedure that is usually uneventful and reluctant to upset their patients with descriptions of postoperative difficulties, medical personnel sometimes imply that the operation is trifling and that recovery is easy. Thus, too many patients hear, "We'll just open your chest, fix your plumbing, and in six weeks, you'll be back on the golf course."

In light of the routine nature of most bypasses, this attitude is understandable. But when you are contemplating surgery or when someone you love is being wheeled to the operating room, the event takes on more imposing proportions. Few people undergo surgery without facing their mortality squarely. Beforehand, nearly all patients and their families feel anxious. Afterwards, patients commonly endure pain and discomfort, lingering weakness, and periodic dejection. Most do not feel like themselves for months. When medical personnel underestimate these physical and emotional difficulties, patients may have trouble reconciling the contradiction between what they hear and what they feel. When this happens, they may experience more physical and emotional pain and take longer to recover than those who know what to expect.

One of the most common difficulties after surgery is depression. The Miami Heart Institute Study, which found that 28% of patients were depressed, suggests that up to 64,000 bypass patients in the United States each year suffer from postsurgical depression. An early study of thirty patients at the University of North Carolina drew

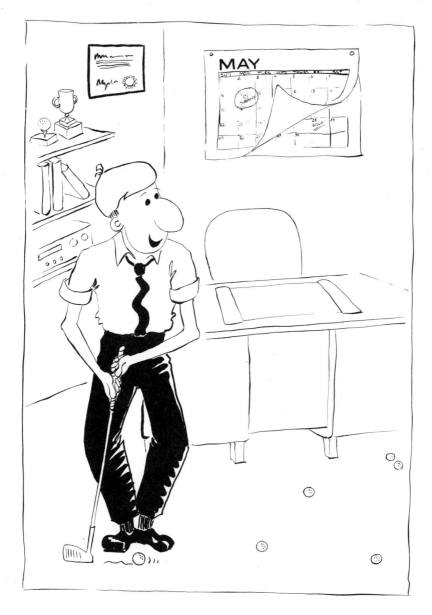

"We'll just open your chest, fix your plumbing,
and in six weeks, you'll be back on the golf course."

similar conclusions. Although surgery was considered successful for all thirty patients, 83% remained unemployed and 57% were sexually impotent up to two years after surgery. These patients reported limited activities, distorted body images, poor self-esteem, and lingering depression. The researchers of this study asserted that the psychological welfare and social adjustment of bypass patients demand more attention. To date, several dozen studies echo the conclusion that while bypass does eradicate or diminish chest pain, many patients are unable to live the fulfilling lives they had anticipated.

As Jonathan Halperin, M.D., Director of Clinical Cardiology at New York's Mount Sinai Medical Center, observes, "Patients are robbed of their sense of well-being or infused with self-doubt. Others cope with the realization of having suddenly grown frail and old . . . . This post-bypass syndrome is taking on the dimensions of a public health problem in its own right."

## The Nature of Crisis and Crisis Intervention

The depression which can afflict heart surgery patients stems largely from the emotional upheaval of the experience. Heart surgery is, after all, a major life crisis. It forces most patients to confront their mortality and harness their fears. Like any other crisis, such as the death of a loved one or an earthquake, heart surgery can impair people's normal ability to cope.

When coping becomes difficult, people stop functioning in their usual ways. They feel overwhelmed and anxious. They have trouble solving problems and setting priorities. The havoc which results makes them feel helpless.

Crisis intervention is counseling designed to enable people to overcome these feelings of helplessness and thereby reduce the additional emotional difficulties that crisis triggers. It is not psychotherapy, not analytical, and not designed to uncover secrets hidden in the unconscious. Nor is it designed to change people. Rather, it is intended to help people anticipate what will happen, understand how they normally cope with crisis, and then mobilize those coping strategies.

Coping styles vary from person to person, and there is no right or wrong style. For example, when a hurricane 500 miles off the coast of Florida seemed to be headed for Miami, Mildred Nerler scurried about bringing in all her potted plants and outdoor furniture. She wanted to be prepared for the worst. Her neighbor thought she was crazy and chose to sit tight until he heard a later forecast.

"Maybe I'll have to scramble at the last minute," he said, "but sure as heck I'm not going to drag all this stuff in for nothing."

Though coping styles are highly personal, everyone usually resorts to the same style time and again. Mildred Nerler does her Christmas shopping in September; her neighbor never starts until the week before the holiday. Long before Mildred Nerler goes on vacation, she begins laying out the clothes she will take. Carefully and unhurriedly, she packs her suitcase, making sure to have it closed and ready the night before her trip. Her neighbor doesn't even begin to think about what he'll take until the night before he leaves. Then, he throws whatever looks clean into a suitcase and hopes he's well prepared. Everyone's responses follow a predictable course, and in a catastrophe people fall back on the strategies they have always found most helpful.

Because people feel overwhelmed and anxious at these times, however, they often have trouble making even their most effective strategies work. One of the goals of counseling is to help people adapt their most reliable strategies to the demands of the trauma. Fortunately, people in crisis seem especially receptive to this therapy.

## Method of the Miami
## Heart Institute Study

To test whether crisis intervention could help heart surgery patients, we provided the following support to half our patients:

Before surgery, our counselors told the patients and their families exactly what events would occur and what sensations and emotions they were likely to feel.

After surgery, counselors gave patients and their families detailed information about the physical and emotional aspects of recovery as well as hospital routine.

The counselors encouraged the nurses, clergy, and family to be supportive.

After discharge, counselors visited each patient and his family at home once a week for eight weeks, by which time the crisis presumablyhad ended and the patients and their families were functioning as usual. These visits were devoted largely to trying to help the family help the patient.

The counselors offered specific suggestions for solving problems pertinent to surgery and recovery, but they avoided becoming involved in extraneous problems, such as stressful family relationships.

To enable us to assess the thoughts, feelings, perceptions, and coping styles of the 104 patients in the study, all of them took nine self-administered psychological tests before surgery. The results of these tests helped the counselors adapt their approach to each patient in the crisis intervention group. Beginning with the first session, the counselors considered each patient's personality and coping style. Some patients took a stoic stance, and counselors listened as they acknowledged, "If I die, I die." Other patients needed reassurance, so counselors listened to their fears and reminded them that, although their fears were understandable, their chances for successful surgery were overwhelmingly in their favor. Many patients, attempting to protect their loved ones, resisted expressing their emotions. The counselors helped these men by listening to them without passing judgment on what they said. Many other patients denied feeling anxious or worried, and the counselors accepted that denial. In most cases, counselors knew, the denial was valuable protection from unbearable fear. Thus, before surgery, counselors accepted whatever feelings the patients expressed without tampering with their defenses. For patients as well as their families, this approach significantly reduced stress.

During hospital visits after surgery, counselors continued to help patients remember important points about their care, which they tended to forget because of stress. Mitchell McCabe, for example, had not slept for the first two days after leaving the intensive care unit (ICU) because he worried his heart would stop and no one would know he was dead. Mitchell McCabe was too anxious to remember he was wearing a heart monitor, so he sat in bed afraid to take his finger off his pulse. When the counselor reminded him of the monitor and explained how it worked, he fell asleep before she finished talking.

Sally Kolitz, one of two counselors who guided the patients and their families through the experience, explained, "My most important role was helping patients anticipate what they would experience physically and emotionally. They appreciated the opportunity to explore their feelings, release them, and understand them. These men also valued hearing that their feelings were normal, that they would end, and that the emotions they were experiencing could legitimately follow physiological and emotional stress."

The majority of patients were stoic, controlled men who had never before confronted their emotions, let alone candidly discussed them with someone else. Yet, in the wake of surgery, some became hyperemotional. In outbursts of rage, they could hurl trays of food on the floor. Some became sentimental and could cry at a situation comedy on television. Understandably, the men and their families were confused and frightened by this uncharacteristic behavior. They made good use of the help which the counselors offered. "Here comes the lady who lets me cry," became a joke among the men.

Nathan Orenstein dramatizes how effectively the counselor's visits eased his emotional pain. From the day this patient left the ICU, he threw every meal tray on the floor. When the nurse brought him a newspaper or magazine, he flung that down as well.

Observing his rage, Sally Kolitz asked, "What's bothering you? What isn't going well?"

Nathan Orenstein listed a host of complaints: the low-salt diet, noise in the halls, inconsiderate nurses, hurried physicians. The counselor commiserated with his plight. Then, suspecting his anger could be an expression of fear, she commented, "In talking to other patients, I find many say that it's scary after surgery. Do you ever have any of these feelings? Do you ever worry what's going to become of you?"

He peremptorily dismissed any such concern. "No, no, I'm going to be just fine."

The counselor dropped the issue for the moment but continued to mention other patients' fears on subsequent visits. Ultimately, this patient let go. Nathan Orenstein was a prominent attorney deeply committed to his work and he secretly anguished that his career was over. The more Nathan Orenstein talked about his fear, the more information the counselor, nurses, and physicians were able to provide. As he received reliable information, his fears diminished.

Had a well-trained counselor not quieted this man's fears, his anger might not have abated. The experience of a patient who did not receive crisis intervention illustrates this point. When Joseph Cobb seemed unreasonably angry, the nurses tried cajoling him. When that approach didn't work, they tried reprimanding him. Being treated like a child only fueled his anger. It never occurred to the nurses that Joseph Cobb was struggling with nagging fears. As his anger intensified, so did the nurses', until they resorted to avoiding him as much as possible. When discharged, Joseph Cobb was still hostile and argumentative, and his wife worried that he had suffered a permanent personality change.

The psychological tests which the patients took before surgery gave us valuable insight into their personalities. By highlighting strengths and vulnerabilities, the profile enabled the physicians, nurses, and counselors to plan the most effective management of each patient. Phillip Raymond's story illustrates this well.

At forty-eight, Phillip Raymond was a brilliant financial analyst who had experienced chest pain on and off for nine years; he was competitive and hard-driving. In addition, he believed he was invincible, and despite recommendations to the contrary, he smoked, ate the wrong foods, remained overweight and sedentary, and avoided his doctor. Ultimately, his chest pain got worse, and he found himself a candidate for bypass surgery.

As one might expect, Phillip Raymond always denied his emotions and kept tight control over all facets of his life. He suffered headaches and stomach pains when he became tense, yet he never acknowledged his concerns even to himself lest he appear weak. Phillip Raymond never complained, not when he worried about his health

and not when he felt sick. He was a perfectionist, sometimes placing impossibly high demands on himself. He
met the ensuing frustration with explosions of temper.
During these moments, he felt the hammer in his head,
the vise grip on his chest, and the knots in his stomach.

To help Phillip Raymond recuperate with minimal
frustration, the medical team capitalized on his need for
control. In the hospital, he became unusually alert to
sensations in his body. His physician responded to his
observations by explaining them at length. Although
Phillip Raymond's hypersensitivity to what he was feeling
could have bred apprehension, the medical team circum-
vented that possibility by giving him the opportunity to
understand his medical condition fully and participate in
planning his rehabilitation.

After surgery, Phillip Raymond healed quickly. Although many patients relinquish some of their denial
after surgery, he did not. He insisted he was fine and
began doing some work from his hospital bed to prove it.
But he became irritable. When the counselor observed
that his angry outbursts stemmed from his need to take
control over his life, the staff went out of their way to let
him make choices and decisions rather than antagonizing
or patronizing him. Yet two problems persisted: his
immersion in his work and his hostile interactions with
his wife and teenage son. To address these problems, the
counselor taught Phillip Raymond some relaxation exercises and discussed his need to reassess his professional
responsibilities. When she talked to the couple, she
invited them to express their respective fears concerning
his surgery and other worries the experience had brought
to light.

Patients like Phillip Raymond often resort to their old
habits as soon as they recover completely. In fact, they
quickly convince themselves that they do not have coronary artery disease and that whatever problem prompted
the surgery no longer exists. Knowing this, the counselor
took advantage of Phillip Raymond's need to control his

life and secured his cooperation in designing some new exercise, relaxation, and eating habits. Predictably, he was resistant at first, but he gradually became aware of worries which he had suppressed. He acknowledged them and began to change. Two years after his surgery, he was still working hard, but he admitted he had always been his own worst enemy and lessened his demands on himself. At the same time, he seemed to grow more tolerant of his family.

## Conclusions of the Study

To some degree, almost all patients in the Miami Heart Institute Study experienced depression, although far fewer in the counseling group were debilitated by it. More significantly, patients in the counseling group seemed better able to recognize depression when it occurred. In contrast, patients who did not receive counseling misunderstood the symptoms of depression. They called their cardiologists and complained of low energy, trouble sleeping, poor appetite, and various discomforts which neither examination nor tests could verify. These symptoms were indicative of depression, not medical difficulties. Crisis intervention, it seems, gave patients in the counseling group enough understanding about themselves and their surgery to identify depression, accept it, and do something constructive about it.

Debilitating depression occurred most frequently among patients who had experienced numerous or significant life changes during the preceding six months and whose surgery entailed many bypasses. Our study suggests that if you fall into one of these categories or if you have periodically experienced depression, you would be wise to arrange for crisis intervention. Otherwise, you probably do not need it.

Even if you are not especially vulnerable, you will probably profit from preparing yourself for surgery in the same way that crisis therapists prepare their patients, and the forthcoming chapters will help. In anticipation of hospitalization, you and your family should know exactly what procedures, physical discomforts, and emotional reactions the experience will entail. You would probably benefit from knowing how others responded at each step, from knowing yourself, and from understanding how you cope best. Inherent in this self-awareness is your understanding of how much control of your life you prefer to take and your ability to adapt this preference to the demands of being a hospital patient.

If you fit the profile of patients prone to postsurgical depression, we urge you to arrange for crisis intervention. Since counseling may keep you away from your cardiologist's office in the future, it is economically prudent as well as practical. We also urge you to select a counselor who is appropriately trained and intuitive enough to be able to provide the special brand of help effective during crisis. He or she should have at least a master's degree in counseling or psychotherapy, know the literature on heart surgery, and have experience working with medical patients. At the very least the professional must be willing to become familiar with the available literature. Your surgeon or cardiologist may be able to recommend a therapist. You can also turn to the psychology or psychiatry department of a local university hospital, the Mental Health Association, the American Heart Association, or a local support group for heart surgery patients.

Crisis intervention is intended to be provided during crisis, not weeks or months afterwards, when reactions can become deeply imbedded. We recommend that you begin as soon as you agree to surgery. Ideally, the therapist would meet with you alone, with your family alone, and with all of you together during several short sessions. In this way, you can all get to know the counselor and grow comfortable talking openly. During hospitalization, you would probably benefit from several short visits with the counselor. After discharge, we recommend weekly sessions in your home and with your family. By the end of about two months, you will probably feel the crisis has been resolved and be ready for the meetings to end.

Should you not elect this kind of therapy from the outset but discover the need for professional help later, do not feel that you have made an irretrievable mistake. While it is preferable to prevent the onset of serious depression, counseling initiated at a later date can help.

Whether or not you need crisis intervention, you would probably benefit from an empathic, loving support system to help you garner your most successful coping strategies. Supporters can provide invaluable help by understanding the feelings you are likely to experience at the various stages of recovery. If your supporters can accept your emotions without feeling threatened, they can help you vent your feelings and restore your perspective.

Gerald Caplan notes that people who successfully weather a crisis emerge more self-confident and better able to cope with future traumas. In other words, difficult experiences hold the potential for growth. If you can utilize the principles of crisis intervention—with or without professional help—you stand to gain more from your surgery than just a healthy heart.

## Points to Remember

Heart surgery can be a major life crisis and leaves one-third of patients suffering from debilitating depression. This depression appears to be aggravated by the inability to cope.

❏ Arrange for crisis intervention to help you cope if you have experienced numerous or significant life changes within six months, if your surgery entails many bypasses, or if you are prone to depression.

❑ Learn what to expect from every facet of recovery.

❑ Understand yourself, how much control over your life you prefer to have, and how you best handle difficult situations.

Chapter Two

# CHOOSING SURGERY

Suddenly you find yourself researching your own prospective heart surgery. Perhaps you thought you were a model of good health until you failed a routine stress test. It is more likely that you have had worrisome chest pain periodically for some time. Maybe you had a heart attack. In any case, your physician is concerned that you are suffering from coronary heart disease. As a result of numerous factors working silently for years—your genes, a diet too high in saturated fats, excessive stress, and smoking, to name some of the possible factors—the arteries which carry blood to your heart muscle have become clogged and cannot deliver blood to it efficiently. This condition may threaten your life.

The heart, like every other organ in the body, needs blood for sustenance. Ironically, although its chambers are filled with blood, the tissues of the muscle itself absorb virtually none of it. Instead, the organ is fed by a system of arteries which branch off the aorta, the main artery carrying freshly oxygenated blood to the smaller arteries and from there throughout the body. (See Appendix II)

When the coronary arteries are healthy, the blood flows through them easily. During exercise or stress, when the heart pumps more quickly and needs additional nourishment, healthy arteries can supply an ample amount of blood. In patients with coronary heart disease, partially blocked arteries can prevent sufficient blood from being delivered to a portion of the muscle. This deprivation usually causes a squeezing sensation in the chest and/or pain in the left arm and perhaps the jaw. Often, this sensation, called angina, lasts only moments. It may come with exercise and stop when the exercise ceases, signaling that sufficient blood flow has been restored. If part of the heart is starved for too long, perma-

21

nent damage occurs; the part of the heart muscle deprived of blood dies and is replaced by scar tissue. This is a heart attack, also called a coronary or a myocardial infarction. It can be fatal if muscle damage is extensive.

Sometimes, the arteries restrict blood to the heart without the telltale symptoms of angina. When this restriction persists, patients may die because they cannot sense that they are having a heart attack and do not get immediate medical attention. Conversely, severe angina or even a heart attack is not necessarily a threat to life. The location and degree of blockages may be more pertinent than pain or minor muscle damage. In some instances, blockages threaten life seriously and must be dealt with surgically. In approximately two-thirds of cases, there are preferable or alternative treatments. The only way to assess coronary artery disease accurately is with a cardiac catheterization.

## Coping with Catheterization

Cardiac catheterization is prescribed when an acute heart attack, intermittent angina, routine stress test, or other studies demand a clear picture of the coronary vessels. Catheterization is the only means for securing this picture and is therefore the ultimate diagnostic test for coronary artery disease. It is also prerequisite to bypass surgery, for it reveals details essential to planning the operation.

Catheterization often requires brief hospitalization; patients are admitted the day before for preliminary tests and observation. Whether the procedure is being performed on an inpatient or outpatient basis, patients are always sedated before they are taken into the catheterization laboratory. In most instances, patients arrive in the lab feeling relaxed, yet alert enough to banter with the professional team and follow the cardiologist's instructions to move, breathe deeply, and cough. The procedure begins when the cardiologist injects a local anesthetic into the inner upper thigh, which has been shaved and scrubbed as it would be for surgery. For most patients, this injection is the most uncomfortable part of the procedure, and it is no more painful than any other injection. Once the area is numb, the cardiologist, guided by an x-ray image of the heart broadcast on a television monitor, inserts a catheter into the femoral artery and threads it to the heart. Since blood vessels are devoid of nerve endings, this part of the procedure is usually sensation free.

Once the catheter is positioned properly in the coronary arteries, the cardiologist injects a contrast medium through the catheter. Usually, as the dye enters the coronary arteries, patients feel suddenly hot. Some patients, prepared for the heat wave, are surprised when they feel virtually nothing. Others agree it was as unpleasant as they were warned it would be. Occasionally, the hot flush is accompanied by an unpleasant fishy taste, an urgent sense of nausea, and vomiting. All these reactions disappear in about sixty seconds.

As the contrast material flows through the heart, it draws a map of the coronary artery system and shows the location and extent of any blockages. It also helps to highlight the mechanical functioning of the heart so that the cardiologist can assess the damage to the muscle as well as the organ's efficiency as a pump. To view the entire heart, the cardiologist repositions the catheter inside the main chamber several times and injects more contrast material each time. With every dose of dye, the heat resurges then subsides. The entire study lasts about one hour, maybe less. Finally, the cardiologist withdraws the catheter—another sensation-free experience—and firm pressure is placed on the artery to prevent bleeding. Although patients must lie still for several hours until the blood has safely clotted, they experience no pain during this time.

When catheterization was initiated in the late 1950s, it seemed an awesome diagnostic tool even to the profes-

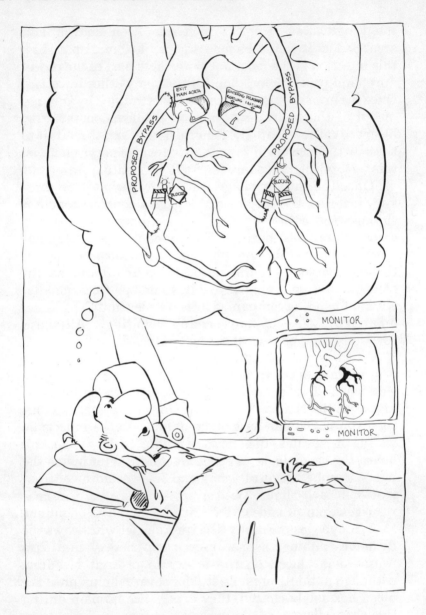

As the contrast material flows through the heart, it draws a map of the coronary artery system and shows the location and extent of any blockages.

sionals who used it. Since then, however, experts have refined the techniques, and the procedure has lost its portentous character as well as most of its attendant risks. Nevertheless, patients often approach the catheterization with trepidation. It is a natural tendency to fear the results, as though the diagnosis would not exist if the catheterization didn't confirm it. For those who have never experienced catheterization before, it also carries the fear of the unknown. Some patients feel invaded and vulnerable. As one woman put it, "The cardiologist literally touched my heart, and there on a television screen, for all the world to see, was my soul." Occasionally, patients even feel threatened by the consent form.

The consent form for cardiac catheterization—like consent for surgery—ensures that you understand the benefits and risks associated with the forthcoming procedure. It also enables the hospital to prove legally that you were appropriately informed. Ideally, your attending physician will discuss with you at length why this procedure is advisable. In candidly disclosing its risks, he or she will tell you that heart attacks, strokes, kidney failure, and a host of other ominous consequences happen on rare occasion, but that in 999 out of 1,000 cases, the procedure is accomplished without any complication whatsoever. Whether you have this discussion with your doctor or a nurse, by the time it is over, you should feel confident that you are having the study because its potential benefits outweigh its risks.

Still, signing the consent form, which lists in painful detail every remote complication, can be frightening. With luck, you will encounter a good nurse, who will help you understand how safe the procedure is. Our nurses mitigated many patients' fears when they emphasized that signing the consent is a formality and that any patient recommended for catheterization was unlikely to encounter a problem. By the same token, a perceptive nurse can quiet patients' apprehension as they wait for the procedure to begin. One man about to undergo catheterization lay in the waiting area worrying about the anesthetic injection he would get in his groin. A nurse asked him why he was worried and when he told her, she responded empathically, "We see lots of folks who are scared of needles." Her acceptance of his feelings together with the sedation helped him to relax, and he managed the procedure without difficulty.

While many patients experience some degree of anxiety before catheterization, some feel none. Some are intrigued by the process and become fascinated watching their hearts on a television screen. And when the procedure is over, nearly everyone is surprised at how easy it really was.

## Deciding on Surgery

Your catheterization may reveal that you have a dangerous blockage of your left main artery. This is the artery that feeds the left ventricle, and the left ventricle is the most important chamber of the heart because it is responsible for pumping oxygen-fresh blood throughout the body. Statistics suggest that, if your left ventricle is deprived of blood, you stand little chance of surviving. Surgery is mandatory and often scheduled within hours.

Statistics also suggest that, if you have more than 70% blockages in three arteries and minor damage to your heart muscle, surgery will lengthen your life. However, if you have triple-vessel disease and a normal heart muscle, it is not clear that surgery will prolong life. For patients in this category and those with other forms of less menacing disease, numerous other considerations come into play. The most important is pain. How intense is your angina? How much does it interfere with your activities?

While surgery has become increasingly safe in recent years, drug therapies have also improved. New medications and new applications of older drugs can successfully compensate for constricted arteries in many patients. These people find that medications eliminate their pain without restricting their lifestyles or endangering their hearts. For other patients, drugs do not solve the problem.

In recent years another option has been developed. This is percutaneous transluminal angioplasty (PCTA). In this procedure, which resembles cardiac catheterization, a balloon is passed through a catheter to the blocked artery. When it reaches the point of occlusion, the balloon is inflated. The resulting pressure widens the coronary artery and restores normal blood flow. Thus, successful transluminal angioplasty accomplishes the same results as bypass surgery with a fraction of the physical or emotional trauma. Recuperation time is reduced to days.

Whether you are a candidate for balloon angioplasty depends on a number of issues, including the number, location, and degree of your blockages and the status of your heart muscle. Approximately one-third of potential bypass patients are good candidates for angioplasty, and for them the procedure is clearly preferable. In the wrong patient, however, angioplasty can lead to emergency bypass surgery, which always carries increased risks.

When angioplasty is inappropriate, surgery may be recommended even if it isn't essential to prolonging life or controlling pain. Some patients, for example, have increasingly frequent angina, which a physician may interpret as a signal of future trouble. On the grounds that an elective procedure is safer than emergency surgery, the physician may recommend bypass before it becomes mandatory. In optional cases, numerous factors affect a physician's thinking. Patients under seventy, for example, statistically do better than older patients, but many older people do exceedingly well. Even certain high-risk patients can benefit significantly from surgery. In some, it can improve the pumping power of the left ventricle, thus increasing the efficiency with which oxygen-rich blood is delivered throughout the body and giving the patient more energy and stamina. Yet the prognosis can also be affected by diabetes, previous heart attacks, degree of damage to the heart muscle, location of the damage, and efficiency of the heart's pumping capability. Chronic lung disease (bronchitis and emphysema, for example) as well as overall health also colors the picture. With so many relevant factors, recommendations for surgery are based as much on judgment as on objective findings.

When surgery is optional, some patients study their conditions so thoroughly that they almost take a postgraduate course in coronary heart disease and its treatments! For example, Jacques Monteil, a fifty-five-year-old Swiss accountant with an insatiable desire for knowledge, read all of the literature he could find, sought additional opinions from recommended specialists, and consulted numerous patients who shared their experiences with him. Patients often seek information because doing so increases their sense of control over their fate. This is not to suggest that everyone should pursue an intensive investigation. The amount and type of information which is helpful varies among people, and you would do well to follow your instincts in deciding what to learn. When information begins to increase anxiety, it may be time to stop learning.

If you want to participate actively in the decision, read *Bypass* by Jonathan Halperin and Richard Levine or *Open Heart Surgery* by Ina Yalof (see Some Additional Resources at the conclusion of this book). Both of these volumes explore the anatomy, physiology, and management of coronary heart disease. After this reading, perhaps you should sit down with the experts and talk specifically about yourself. While statistics about risks and prognosis offer valuable guidelines, you are not a statistic; you are a person with a unique health history as well as unique physiological and psychological dynamics.

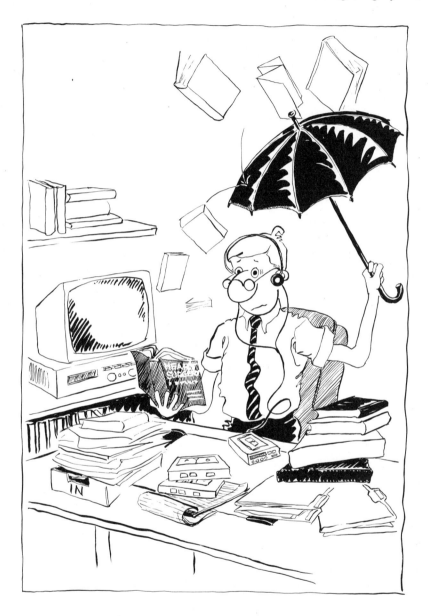

When surgery is optional, some patients study their conditions so
thoroughly that they almost take a postgraduate course in
coronary heart disease and its treatments!

Since recommendations for surgery often rely heavily on a physician's judgment and perception, it's not unlikely for experts to disagree, as journalist Douglass Cater discovered. Douglass Cater, who chronicled his valve replacement surgery in a *New York Times Magazine* article entitled "How to Have Open-Heart Surgery (and Almost Love It)," acknowledged that he encountered his greatest difficulties when he tried to reconcile conflicting opinions among physicians he respected. Yet he found the act of deciding to have surgery invigorating.

When Jacques Monteil investigated the advisability of surgery, he consulted two specialists and asked each these questions:

*Why is bypass surgery better for me than medication?*

*Can my arteries be repaired using a less invasive technique? Am I a candidate for transluminal (balloon) angioplasty?*

*Presuming I am not a good candidate for balloon angioplasty, what factors make me a good candidate for bypass surgery? What factors stand as potential obstacles? How are the risks balanced against the benefits?*

*If I agree to bypass surgery, what are my chances for success in light of my unique health circumstances?*

*Exactly what does success mean for me? Specifically, how will surgery alter the quality of my life?*

*How long are the benefits of surgery likely to last?*

*What is involved in the surgery and recovery? What problems can the heart-lung machine cause and what is the likelihood that residual difficulties will affect my lifestyle?* (The heart-lung machine takes over respiration and circulation while the coronary arteries are being repaired. Although this machine is an effective substitute for the heart and lungs during surgery, its use has occasionally been implicated in postsurgical neurological difficulties. In the vast majority of cases, these problems are minor and transient.)

*Would you create the bypasses using the saphenous vein from the leg, the mammary artery from the chest wall, or both?* (In general, the saphenous vein is easier to extract but may become clogged with atherosclerotic plaque more quickly than the mammary artery. Other factors relevant to your particular case will undoubtedly contribute to your surgeon's choice in this regard.)

Although Jacques Monteil's angiogram showed several severe blockages, the two specialists he consulted disagreed about whether he should have surgery. Jacques Monteil sought the advice of a third expert, whose opinion both the others respected. This consultant advised surgery, but Jacques Monteil was still not ready to make the commitment. First he wanted to talk to some friends and acquaintances who had undergone the procedure. He wrote in the journal he kept throughout the experience:

> [They] told me about the relief that the operation had brought them and the fact that it had changed their lives. Man doesn't like to live with a sword of Damocles over his head, so after a couple of months of hard thinking, I decided to go ahead with the surgery.

Bypass surgery is not for everyone. Personality and way of life affect the decision. Some patients prefer taking medication to confronting the risk of a surgically induced heart attack or stroke, even though this risk ranges from a low of 1/2% in younger candidates to only 3% in older candidates. One patient explained her refusal to have surgery this way: "You're alive or you're dead, and when it's you, statistics don't mean one single thing."

Feeling this way made forty-seven-year-old Donald Lawford resist surgery initially. He had first experienced chest pain while jogging. After appropriate testing, his cardiologist recommended surgery, but Donald Lawford wanted to try medication first and switched to a doctor who was willing to go along with him. For a while, medications which the new physician prescribed controlled his pain, but before long, Donald Lawford was experiencing angina whenever he walked. When he was hospitalized to prevent a coronary, he underwent another stress test, which confirmed his illness. At that point, the new cardiologist ordered a cardiac catheterization and, after reviewing it, recommended surgery.

He said, "We tried medication and it didn't work. Given your blockages you will probably have a fatal coronary."

When faced with that alternative, Donald Lawford agreed to surgery. He liked the way this physician approached his illness one step at a time. What Donald Lawford perceived as a logical, conservative approach helped him accept the physician's recommendation for surgery and go into it with a positive attitude.

"If I had been railroaded into surgery, I would have always wondered if there was some other alternative that would have been adequate."

Some patients who choose medication initially change their minds because they cannot tolerate the steady reminders that they are ill. Ivan Kolnikow, for example, tried nitroglycerine for three months when he was first given a choice. Though he was bothered by gripping chest pains from time to time, his tests showed that his two blockages were not life-threatening, and he was in no rush to have surgery.

"After a while, I couldn't stand this angina. I never knew when it would get me. It was like a shadow always over my shoulder. Finally I decided: Either I'll live like a whole person or to hell with it."

Other patients for whom surgery is optional take this view immediately. They cannot bear to perceive themselves as ill. Risk or no, they choose surgery feeling that they want to live vigorously or die. Even some high-risk patients feel this way. As one patient admitted, "My cardiologist told me I had a terrible disease and I know I'm going into surgery with no guarantees. But I'm certainly not going to feel good without the operation, so I'll roll the dice."

For patients who passionately embrace vigorous activities, surgery is worth its physical, emotional, and financial costs. "It's a second chance, a new life," said one former patient. And he should know. After two heart attacks, he could barely walk around the block. Now he runs, pedals his ten-speed bike over hilly terrain, lifts weights, and, at age seventy-two, just got married for the first time. Like this reborn septuagenarian, most bypass patients emerge from surgery liberated from the clenches of angina and free, often for the first time in years, to walk, sail, or ski the Rockies.

## Choosing a Surgeon

It is important for all patients wheeled into the operating room to believe that surgery is the best treatment for their disease and that they are in the very best professional hands. Many people have no trouble acquiring trust and taking their internist's or cardiologist's recommendation for a surgeon. As one patient put it, "My gut feeling was this guy was good, and that was enough for me." He did not feel comfortable interrogating a prospective physician. If anything, the idea of planning the investigation and sorting out conflicting recommendations made him dizzy.

Other people feel uncomfortable putting themselves in the hands of a professional until they satisfy themselves that they have made the best possible choice. Thus, another patient checked his surgeon's credentials in the library, visited his surgeon's hospital, and talked to patients as well as staff. He looked into the ratio of nurses to patients, the role of aides, and the staff's reputation for delivering sensitive, caring attention. Only after this tenacious research did he feel he was making a decision he could trust.

No matter how dedicated to research you are, it is exceedingly difficult to choose a surgeon independently unless you have a sophisticated medical background. If you feel compelled to participate in the decision, select someone who, at the very least, is a board-certified thoracic surgeon. Certification verifies the surgeon's training and knowledge. You can check physicians' credentials in Marquis' *Directory of Medical Specialties* or the American Board of Medical Specialties' *Compendium of Certified Medical Specialists*. Both of these multivolume directories, available at many public libraries, list more than 300,000 board-certified specialists according to specialty and location. Both include the physicians' ages, where they trained, what certifications they hold, when they were certified, and what hospitals they use. The Marquis publication also summarizes the physicians' careers and thus sheds additional light on their experience.

Where physicians trained and the experts they trained under are important. Look for prominent hospitals with highly reputed heart surgery departments and renowned senior surgeons. In addition, select a surgeon whose performance record compares favorably with national statistics. Nationwide, fewer than three patients in 100 suffer serious complication or death from bypass surgery.

Can the surgeon you are considering claim the same? If the answer is yes, particularly if this surgeon operates on high-risk patients, he or she is probably a good choice. Before making a commitment, however, you would be wise to ask these questions:

*How many procedures do you perform in a day? In a week?* (It's important for surgeons to operate swiftly but accurately, especially when patients are on the heart-lung machine. The less time patients are on this machine, the better. When patients are on the machine for longer than two hours, the risk of postoperative problems rises significantly. To operate efficiently, surgeons must stay well practiced. They must do enough procedures in a week to keep their skills honed but not so many in one day that they become fatigued.)

*How many procedures in a week does your team perform together? With you? With other surgeons?* (For surgery to progress efficiently, the team must work in perfect synchrony. When a team works together often, they mesh with one another like a set of well-matched gears, and they speed the surgery along.)

Since it is so difficult for a novice to select a surgeon, referrals from knowledgeable people can be invaluable. Your cardiologist is probably the best person to advise you. If you ask several physicians and the same recommendation comes up repeatedly, it's probably a good one. Some people say knowledgeable, forthright nurses are the best source for professional recommendations, and usually referrals from professionals are more reliable than recommendations from lay people. In any case, it is important to evaluate the source of the recommendation and treat the advice accordingly.

Some patients are content when they feel that they have chosen the best trained, most highly regarded surgeon available. They never stop to consider the surgeon's personality. One patient, who values his vitality more than his life, insisted it would never occur to him to investigate a surgeon's bedside manner: "I don't care if he's the meanest, most insensitive son of a so-and-so who ever furrowed a mother's brow. Just make sure he's a genius with a knife, and let his wife worry about his personality."

For other patients, however, a surgeon's bedside manner is very important. In fact, one of the most frequent complaints of bypass patients is that their surgeons neglected them during the postoperative period. Some patients complained they never saw their surgeons after they woke up from anesthesia. More frequently, patients were frustrated because they felt their surgeons' visits, though regular, were perfunctory. While these patients hoped their surgeons would sit down, listen to their hearts, and spend a few unhurried minutes talking and answering questions, the surgeons poked their heads in the door, said something like, "Just checked your chart. Glad to see everything is going well," and disappeared before the patients could formulate a question.

Undoubtedly there are many reasons for this problem. To be sure, heart surgeons are busy and rarely have time for chatting. Patients recovering from surgery, on the other hand, have more time and are more preoccupied with themselves than usual. The brevity of the surgeons' visits may seem exaggerated by contrast. To exacerbate this problem, many surgeons consider bypass surgery commonplace. Happily, most bypass procedures are uneventful, and after performing thousands of such operations and watching patients follow a predictable course of recovery, surgeons sometimes forget how important this event is to each patient. Unforgivable though that callousness might seem, in a perverse way it is reassuring.

In addition, many surgeons are better at operating than at communicating and chose their specialty in part because they are more at ease when their patients are anesthetized.  Even those who enjoy spending time talking with their patients sometimes avoid it lest they get too involved.  As Tufts University professor of psychiatry Richard Blacher, M.D., explained, "The pressures of taking scalpel to body and exploring and even seeming to mutilate the very person he is trying to help may make [the surgeon] hesitate to know the patient too intimately."

Regardless of the reason, the problem is a reality, and if you feel lengthy daily visits with your surgeon are imperative, you should try to assess your surgeon's pattern in this regard.  At the same time, since some of the best surgeons are not personable, you may need to compensate.  Your cardiologist, your surgeon's physician's assistant, a clinical nurse specialist, psychological counselor, or patient educator will visit regularly, answer questions competently and patiently, and thereby assuage your concerns.

## Choosing a Hospital

While many experts contend that the choice of surgeon is more important than the choice of hospital, others believe just the opposite.  Regardless of which you select first, hospital and surgeon go hand in hand to some extent because every surgeon admits patients only to certain hospitals.  Often, selecting your hospital is another area where you can exercise some control.

Is the hospital you are considering staffed by nurses and technicians who have been specially trained to meet the needs of heart surgery patients?  Is the hospital equipped with state-of-the-art technology, which can dramatically improve the safety of surgery? (For example, a pulse oximeter, used while patients are anesthetized, warns when patients' oxygen levels fall dangerously low before the deficit can cause irreversible damage. A carbon dioxide capnograph also provides critical information for the anesthesiologist. By graphically representing the carbon dioxide being exhaled, this device reveals how anesthesia is affecting the patients' metabolism. It thus aids the anesthesiologist in the same way that flight instruments guide pilots through storms. These and other sophisticated monitors and machinery can make the difference between successful and unsuccessful surgery.)

Beyond these primary criteria, there are other important factors to consider: Would you prefer a city hospital, where experience is broad but care may be impersonal, or a private hospital, where the opposite may be true? A teaching hospital, where the staff is likely to be aware of the latest research and newest technology, where a house staff — for better or for worse — is on call twenty-four hours a day, seven days a week, and where each patient is likely to be the subject of study, discussion, and probing designed as much for the students' benefit as the patient's? Or a non-teaching hospital, where physicians' assistants may be the most highly trained professionals immediately available? There are pros and cons for each, and the records of individual hospitals, together with their respective professionals and facilities, warrant investigation.

It is always a good idea to ask your physicians which hospital they would choose and why if they were the patients. Unquestionably, cardiologists and surgeons know the various hospitals intimately and have a preference. If you are persistent, you can usually get even the most reluctant physician to reveal it.

In addition, hospital procedures and regulations vary, and all other things being equal, you may make your choices based on these details. For example, in some hospitals, families cannot visit patients once they have been sedated for surgery or while they are in ICU. In some hospitals, patients can have all their blood tests, chest x-rays, and other preoperative studies performed on an outpatient basis. They can even spend the night before surgery out of the hospital, walk into the hospital the morning of surgery, and have their families with them until they go into the operating room. However, most surgeons insist that, because of the seriousness of heart surgery, patients must spend at least one night before surgery as inpatients under medical supervision.

## Choosing a Cardiologist

Even though you are in the hospital for surgery, most surgeons would want you to be seen regularly by a cardiologist. This physician, whose interests are internal medicine and diseases of the heart, serves as quarterback of the medical team. It is the cardiologist's job, for example, to make sure that medications the surgeon prescribes for your heart ·don't conflict with different medications you are taking for an unrelated condition. The cardiologist maintains an overview of you as a whole patient while the surgeon, anesthesiologist, and other specialists concentrate on specific areas. With his broad perspective, the cardiologist balances the narrow focus of each specialist; he makes sure that their respective efforts are properly coordinated and double-checks for omissions and errors. The cardiologist is also likely to assume the role of your advocate, to visit leisurely each day, answer questions, and solve problems.

Ideally, you already have a cardiologist with whom you have established rapport. If you don't or if your cardiologist does not have privileges in the hospital where your surgeon operates, you may have to select one. Your internist or surgeon is a good person to make a recommendation. Left on your own, you should choose an internist who is board-certified in the subspecialty of cardiology and who has been elected a Fellow of the American College of Cardiology, an honorary organization recognizing outstanding practitioners. This physician should also have experience at a prominent hospital with a well-reputed heart surgery department.

## Choosing an Anesthesiologist

Professionals often assert that the anesthesiologist is the most critical person on the surgery team, yet traditionally, this is one area where patients are given no choice. Usually, patients don't even know who their anesthesiologist will be until this mystery person stops in to visit the night before surgery. However, if you are so inclined, you can try to learn about your hospital's anesthesiologists and participate in the choice.

When professionals evaluate an anesthesiologist, they consider his or her judgment and track record. With today's anesthetic techniques, patients receive the desired anesthetic effects with a minimum of risk; they can be asleep, feel no pain, and be subjected to less toxicity than former techniques allowed. But the new techniques demand that a number of anesthetic agents be administered meticulously and that patients be monitored scrupulously.

Each patient is put to sleep by several drugs given intravenously. Once the patient is unconscious, the anesthesiologist inserts an endotracheal tube, which provides an unobstructed channel for the passage of gases and which keeps oral and gastric contents from entering the lungs. This tube is inserted into the patient's mouth, down the throat, between the vocal cords, and into the windpipe. At the moment when the endotracheal tube is put in place, patients are vulnerable and the procedure must be completed in less than one minute. To confound this challenge, anatomic idiosyncrasies, which the anesthesiologist cannot discover until the intubation is underway, occasionally make the maneuver particularly difficult.

Maintaining the ideal balance of drugs is also difficult. Consequently, patients are occasionally anesthetized enough to feel no pain but remain conscious enough to hear the surgeon and nurses faintly. This problem is not serious, but patients find it distressing. In other rare instances, patients regain consciousness before all the effects of the drugs which immobilize the muscles for the surgeon have worn off. Again, this problem is not dangerous, though it can be frightening. Both these occurrences illustrate the complexity of the anesthesiologist's tasks.

Since the anesthesiologist's job is so critical, many patients go into surgery with increased confidence when they have had a say in choosing their anesthesiologist. Moreover, while anesthesiologists often cannot avoid scratching the throat, straining the jaw, or chipping a tooth, patients sometimes hope that by participating in the choice, they will find an anesthesiologist who is particularly gentle.

When asked to recommend an anesthesiologist, surgeons commonly reply, "Everyone on our staff is first-rate." This may be true, and all anesthesiologists may have a fine record where serious complications are concerned. Nevertheless, as surgeons and operating room nurses often confide, if they were patients, they would be sure to choose a specific one or two anesthesiologists from among that first-rate staff.

In choosing an anesthesiologist, consider the following:

*Is he or she board-certified?*

*How often does he work with bypass surgery?*

*How long has he been at your hospital?*

*How often does he work with your team?*

*How well is he respected and trusted by other physicians and hospital staff?*

*Does he take time to explain what he will do?*

*Has he been guilty of malpractice?*

*Does he see his patients after surgery?* (This is a clue to how much he cares.)

One patient, about to undergo surgery in a distant city, called a physician friend long distance to discuss his fears about anesthesia. The friend suggested, "Ask your surgeon who would be his anesthesiologist if he were the patient. When he gives you the party line, press him. Tell him you're sure they are all fine but that he would have a preference anyway. What would his preference be? He'll probably answer you honestly."

The patient followed his friend's advice. His surgeon responded as the friend had predicted. And the patient went into surgery feeling confident that he had the best possible anesthesiologist.

## Banking Your Own Blood

Despite careful scrutiny and reliable tests for AIDS and hepatitis, there is still a remote risk of contracting these diseases through blood transfusions. In an attempt to protect their patients, most hospitals doing heart surgery have taken a number of steps to reduce the need to transfuse patients with blood of strangers.

If your operation is elective, you can probably bank a pint or two of your own blood, all you are likely to need. To bank two pints, begin three weeks before surgery. If you give one pint then and another two weeks later, your body will have plenty of time to replenish its loss. If you cannot bank your own blood, family members whose type matches yours can donate blood and have it designated for your use.

Once 75% of patients lost enough blood to require transfusions during and immediately after surgery. However, with the advent of cell-saver technology, blood lost during surgery and the early postoperative hours can be recaptured, processed, filtered, and returned to the patient. This technology reduces the number of patients needing transfusions by about 40%.

## Points to Remember

❑ Go into surgery understanding how you will benefit from it and believing you are in good hands.

❑ Ask questions and seek enough information to feel confident of a good surgical outcome.

❑ As soon as you agree to surgery, inquire about banking your own blood or having your family bank blood for you.

Chapter Three
# GETTING READY FOR SURGERY

People differ in their feelings about being a hospital patient. Some equate self-esteem and dignity with the control they maintain over their lives, and the passive role of hospital patient conflicts with the self-reliance they prefer. Every facet of the hospital experience heightens their feelings of dehumanizing dependence. These patients manage hospitalization best when they can participate directly in their care and maintain as much control as possible. In contrast, others feel comforted by the patient role and feel secure relinquishing decisions and choices to others; they feel reassured by the promise that someone else will take care of them. "Put me to sleep, do what you want, and wake me when it's over," they would likely say. All patients and their instincts for control fall somewhere between these two extremes. If you can approach hospitalization in a way that suits your needs in this regard, you stand a good chance of managing the experience successfully.

One of the ways hospitals help patients maintain control is by introducing them to the experiences they will encounter. At some hospitals, patients tour the operating room and surgical intensive care unit. They see patients newly out of surgery with all their tubes still in place. Then they visit someone whose surgery took place the day before to witness the progress that occurs in less than twenty-four hours. While nothing can be more reassuring than seeing someone one day after surgery sitting up in bed with no visible tubing except an oxygen cannula, some hospitals are reluctant to subject their ICU patients to this indignity. They resort instead to films or descriptions from nurses trained as patient educators.

## Patient Education

Good patient education includes a description of procedures before and during surgery as well as the sensations patients experience afterwards. Many hospitals encourage family members to participate in these sessions in an attempt to reduce their anxiety, encourage communication between patient and loved ones, and thereby foster mutual support. Patients often find that attending patient education classes with their families reduces their sense of isolation.

"After the film, my wife and I talked about what we had seen. It felt so good to have something to talk about. Somehow, the stress each of us was feeling made talking about anything hard. The film broke the ice," one patient recalled.

Talking about the class later helped another couple to clarify what each had misunderstood and enabled them to formulate questions to ask the patient educator when she visited them privately.

"When questions are generated this way, people get a good, solid sense of what's going on. It helps them to ask questions they might think are silly, and, believe me, there are no silly questions in this business. It also helps them to verbalize vague concerns," the patient educator observed.

While spelling out procedures and sensations is important, the key component of good patient education is teaching several important skills which you will need to perform after surgery to promote recovery. If you practice these exercises until they become routine before surgery, you will perform them more effectively afterwards. Consequently, you are likely to recover more quickly and need less pain medication than you otherwise would.

Much of the work you will have to do after surgery is designed to undo the effects of general anesthesia, which congests and shrinks the lungs. To expand them, loosen and release secretions, and thereby prevent pneumonia, you must begin breathing deeply and coughing soon after your operation. Normally, you wouldn't give these activities a second thought. But with a new chest incision, coughing and breathing are painful and make you feel as if your incision will break open. This cannot happen. Nevertheless, you should learn the techniques which will enable you to clear your lungs productively with a minimum of discomfort.

First you will need to support, or "splint," your rib cage to reduce the pain which accompanies the lung exercises. This is done by hugging a stiff pillow. Since ordinary bed pillows are too soft for effective support, some hospitals provide special ones for this purpose. Other hospitals hand out specially designed teddy bears. Squarish and firm, these foot-tall cuddly creatures afford perfect support for the chest wound. In addition, they wordlessly convey a message of commiseration and emotional support.

"They're a great hit around here," noted Barbara Friedman, clinical nurse specialist in cardiothoracic surgery at Florida's North Ridge Medical Center. "Even our toughest men patients come to love them, though they're sometimes embarrassed to take them at first. It's not unusual to see these guys lying in bed holding the bear. And everybody takes them home."

To practice the deep breathing exercise, take a good, stiff pillow or suitable stuffed animal, place it against your chest, and hug it tightly with both arms. With the pillow in place, inhale through your nose and exhale through your mouth twice, watching your abdomen rise and fall each time. Then inhale, hold your breath for two seconds, and cough twice.

Sitting up with a new chest incision will also be easier if you practice the following technique before surgery: To get out of the left side of the bed, roll onto your left side and

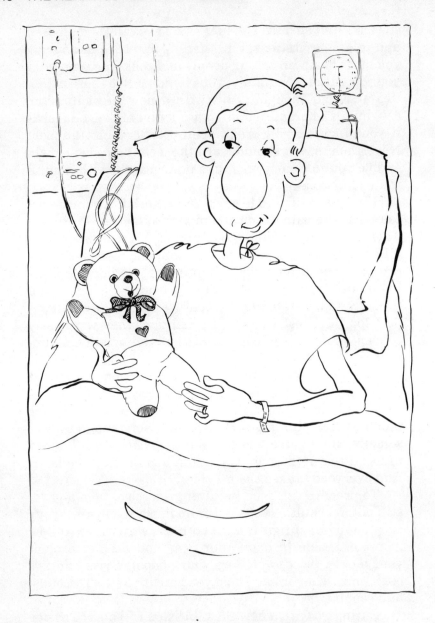

"Even our toughest men patients come to love them,
though they're sometimes embarrassed to take them at first."

pivot your legs so they form an L with your body. Placing your top hand on the bed, use that hand to push yourself up. At the same time, drop your legs over the edge of the bed.

In addition to these exercises, some patients practice relaxation exercises and mantras of positive thoughts to help them manage their most difficult moments. Book stores and libraries offer many volumes and tapes detailing the how-to of Zen philosophies, meditation, and self-hypnosis. Joseph R. Feist, Ph.D., notes that people respond differently to different kinds of relaxation exercise, and he suggests a variety, which you may have to modify slightly to accommodate postoperative discomfort. If you find one or several which soothe you, use them to sustain a state of relaxation for fifteen or twenty minutes.

*1. Lying on your back, tense your feet and relax them. Squeeze and let go; squeeze and let go. Then tense and relax your leg muscles three times. In a similar fashion, tense and relax each muscle group one at a time until you have consciously relaxed your whole body. Then try to sustain a state of utter relaxation.*

*2. Choose a single word, such as "one." While concentrating on breathing slowly, regularly, and deeply, repeat this word every time you exhale. One . . . one . . . one.*

*3. While breathing slowly and regularly, imagine you are blowing away anxiety each time you exhale. Out it goes. It rises up, up, up; it dissipates and disappears.*

*4. Imagine you are in a beautiful, peaceful place.*

*You are drifting in a rowboat on a calm blue lake. You are lying on soft grass beneath the soothing sun of a May afternoon. You are quiet. You are safe.*

*5. Imagine a series of appealing thoughts: A tropical rain forest dense with dewy green; the cheeping of birds, high in the pines of a Maine forest; the sweet fragrance of lilacs; the taste of ice cream, smooth and cold.*

Some patients also find that repeating positive statements eases their distress before surgery and afterwards. Here are some you might try:

*I am having surgery because it will give me a better life than I could have without it.*

*My physician believes I can recover.*

*I may feel frightened (or worried or sad) now, but these feelings will go away.*

*My strength will return. I will get better.*

## Preoperative Procedures

In addition to learning about surgery, you should expect a busy, sometimes annoying routine in the day or two before your operation. The exact sequence of events varies among hospitals and depends, in part, on what time of day your surgery is scheduled.

After blood tests, x-rays, and other laboratory work, you will probably be given an enema. You will take a shower with an antibacterial cleanser and will be shaved from neck to feet. Before you leave your room for surgery, you will be asked to divest yourself of jewelry (though some hospitals agree to tape wedding bands in place), glasses, and hairpieces. Women may be asked to take off their nail polish and makeup so that the physicians can monitor the color of their lips and nail beds. In the operating room, just before administering sleep-inducing drugs, the anesthesiologist will ask you to take out any dentures or removable bridges, which will be returned in the ICU. This preparation can feel terribly degrading.

At some point, usually the day or evening before surgery, the surgeon, cardiologist, and various other staff people will stop by to visit, describe their roles, and ask questions pertinent to their duties. Some will perform a physical exam. Patients often find it bothersome to answer the same questions repeatedly and submit to the same poking by various pairs of hands. "Why can't I talk once and be examined once, and let the other doctors get their information in conference?" one might reasonably ask. Here's the answer: Each physician takes his or her own history and performs her own examination because someone else's written answers prevent her from hearing *how* the patient answers a specific question, which is often as revealing as the answer itself. Furthermore, each physician considers answers to those same questions and approaches physical examination from a different point of view. In turn, any one answer or finding may lead to additional queries, which may have relevance to one specialty, but not to another.

If you have arranged for crisis intervention therapy, the counselor will join the parade. You will also meet your anesthesiologist, who will explain his or her tasks, the drugs they involve, and the postoperative sensations they provoke. During this visit it is important to tell the anesthesiologist about all crowns, bridges, and other permanent dental restorations as well as any eye problems, past or present.

Take advantage of the various presurgical visits to run through all your questions and discuss all your concerns.

While the patient education sessions answer many questions, answers invariably prompt new questions; this is an ideal time to ask them. Just as every physician asks the same questions during a medical history, some patients like to ask every doctor the same questions, in part for reassurance and in part to enlarge their perspective. Even though each answer to a given question may say essentially the same thing, the nuances and points of emphasis are likely to vary. It's a good idea to keep a note pad handy to jot down questions as they crop up and to keep track of key points of the answers; the stress inherent in the preoperative period tends to make concentrating and remembering difficult.

## Emotions before Surgery

By the time you reach this point in the bypass experience, you will probably have confronted the special emotional significance implicit in surgery to the heart. Culturally, the heart is the home of the soul. Though emotions are actually born in the brain, we speak as though love, pain, courage, and hatred emanate from the heart. Jilted lovers suffer from broken hearts. Cold and callous people have hearts of stone. Candor comes forth in heart-to-heart talks. Children "cross their hearts and hope to die" when they seal a promise, and adults vow their sincerity saying, "I mean it with all my heart." In virtually every culture from prehistoric times, the heart has been synonymous with life and feeling.

Actually, the heart is just one of several vital organs. In fact, the heart can often withstand surgery with considerably less risk than, say, the pancreas or the liver. Bypass surgery, for example, usually carries no more than a 3% risk—astonishing news to patients who assume their chances for survival are fifty-fifty. Moreover, with successful transplants and temporary reliance on artificial hearts, there are more treatment options for terminal cardiovascular disease than for diseases of some other vital organs. These truths do not diminish the heart's mystical significance, however. And characteristically, patients perceive the period during surgery when their hearts lie still as temporary death.

Ned Day spoke for many patients when he insisted, "You're dead for a while. While you're on the heart-lung machine, you're dead."

Thinking this way, some patients expect to visit their loved ones in heaven. Some go so far as to face a real conflict: Should they come back or not? Some worry that, once they've seen heaven, they won't want to. Others worry they won't be able to. And occasionally patients emerge from surgery with reports of out-of-body experiences. These are normal responses, and although they are far from universal, they attest to the awe which the prospect of heart surgery carries.

Approaching surgery, some patients seem to have their emotions all worked out. Even a patient with a lifelong dread of blood and needles was able to say that he was more afraid not to have bypass and suffer the consequences than face his fears and go forward. Patients like this have apprehension under control, place complete confidence in their physicians, and enter surgery with philosophical resignation: "If I have to have surgery, so be it."

In contrast, other patients are struck with disbelief. "Me? Bypass surgery? Here I am lying in the hospital, and I still can't believe it."

Often, patients feel intense anger. Some, particularly men who were raised believing that fear is a sign of weakness, express their fear as anger in a variety of ways. One patient, whose surgery was postponed twice, became increasingly agitated, as if the very act of waiting eroded his patience. Other patients complain about the medical personnel, the hospital, or the state of the world in general. Patients may blame themselves for needing surgery.

Their tempers may explode unreasonably at the people they love; probably, they're angry at heart disease or at their predicament. They may, on some level, feel angry at the medical personnel because they delivered the bad news. If so, they're unlikely to vent their fury at these people whose care they need, and they misdirect it toward those they love most. Because patients trust the love of their family and close friends, they unconsciously make them a target for undeserved anger. "Why are you late? Why did you come so early? Why can't you appreciate the way I feel? Why are you patronizing me?" Some patients make their loved ones feel as though they can't do anything right.

Although each patient approaches surgery with a unique emotional portrait, to some extent all patients experience anxiety. Many worry most about relinquishing their self-control. Others dread postoperative pain in the chest and leg. And some fear they will die. Some become introspective and pensive; though they may not verbalize their concerns, what they say and do confirms they are confronting their mortality. They make wills if they don't have them, review their lives, evaluate their accomplishments, and think about the people who have played significant roles over the years. Many patients are openly frightened. As one said, "People do die. You've got to be stupid not to wonder whether you'll ever kiss your wife again." Many, however, manage their anxiety privately. Some, mostly men who were trained from childhood to equate courage and self-reliance with stoicism, preserve their dignity by worrying in silence. Afterwards they sometimes admit that silence was painful. If they found themselves in the same position again, they would try to be open about their feelings.

"I've never been good at talking about feelings," one man acknowledged. "Men like to talk about things. Feelings don't fit into words and make me feel uncomfortable. But there I was in the hospital bed. I'm looking at my wife and wondering, are we ever gonna sleep together again? She's looking at me and she's trying to smile, but her lip is shaking. I'm not saying anything and she's not saying anything. I think it would have been easier for both of us if I could've said . . . you know . . . I tried to pretend I wasn't scared, but I didn't convince either of us."

For some patients, a sense of loneliness pervades, especially at night.

"I'd close my eyes, and I'd see the same vision in my head. It was night and I was alone in my car trapped on a one-way street jammed with traffic. Slowly, slowly I was propelled closer to the black tunnel at the end of the road. I could see it. I didn't want to go into it. But some force stronger than I was kept pushing me forward. Then I'd open my eyes and I'd be in this damned bed. I felt so alone and frightened I almost wished morning would come. And yet I was terrified because I knew it would."

Fear of this kind, painful though it is, can be very helpful. Dr. Irving Janis, author of *Psychological Stress,* found that patients who displayed a moderate amount of anticipatory fear before surgery appeared to have the best outcome. These patients tend to ask questions about their surgery and rehearse the physical and emotional experiences they will encounter. In Irving Janis' words, this "work of worrying" serves as "emotional inoculation" to prepare patients to cope.

Michael Strickland, a thirty-five-year-old insurance broker, worked at worrying for the three weeks between his catheterization and his surgery. During brief bouts with apprehension, his heart pounded and butterflies fluttered in his stomach. The evening before surgery, the hospital counselor talked with him and listened to his fears. Despite his anxiety beforehand, Michael Strickland had no trouble after his operation. He was out of the intensive care unit in two days and recovered quickly.

Because the heart carries unique mystical significance, heart surgery can prompt a unique sequence of emotions. Psychiatrist Richard Blacher, in *The Psychological Experience of Surgery*, summarizes a study comparing the anxiety levels of general surgical patients to those of heart surgery patients. Patients in both groups took psychological tests to measure their apprehension before and after their operations and the general surgery patients, almost universally, registered dramatically high levels of anxiety, which fell sharply during recuperation. For many heart surgery patients, just the reverse was true. Although most of these patients encountered apprehension at some point before their procedures, it miraculously disappeared the day before. Richard Blacher hypothesizes that because of the awesome nature of heart surgery, most patients instinctively resort to denial to protect them from fear. If this theory is valid, then the apprehension which bypass patients sometimes experience after surgery can be explained as a delayed reaction, similar to the nervousness which someone perilously close to an accident experiences after the danger has passed.

Compared to the anguish which Michael Strickland felt, the relief from anxiety which patients often experience the day before can be wonderful. One patient, who had his first heart attack ten years earlier and then endured a second followed by increasing angina, claimed he felt no apprehension whatever going into the operation. "I did not let this get to me at all. I didn't want my sons to think I was falling apart. It was important to show strength to my family," he said, adding that he reassured his family as he was wheeled into the operating room. "I was concerned, yes. Scared, no. Surgery had to be done, so I did it."

Another patient denied ever worrying. Although he acknowledged that patients sometimes die and that the operation is serious, he did not review his will or his life insurance policies. He presumed from the outset that he would survive, recover quickly, and return to work.

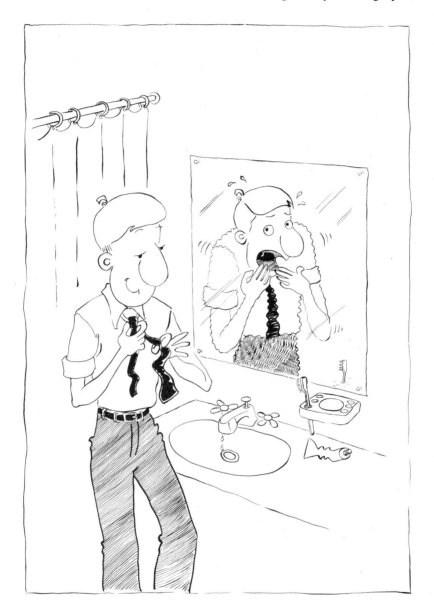

Most patients instinctively resort to denial to protect them from fear.

A third patient acknowledged momentary misgivings, especially after his patient education class. But, he claimed these misgivings vanished quickly. He preferred not to see his family the morning of surgery and went single-mindedly forward.

Journalist Douglass Cater tried hard to draw the curtain of denial over his fear the night before surgery, but he was not entirely successful, so he turned instead to dictating a message of farewell into his tape recorder, just in case. Later, he described his feelings during these dark moments: "It's an awkward exercise and by the time I have finished, I find there is a painful lump in my throat. Somewhat akin to Tom Sawyer's participation in his own funeral."

Some patients deal with their anxieties by forcing themselves to ignore information that frightens them. They don't want to know what experiences to expect. They don't want to go to the patient education classes. Douglass Cater purposely avoided reading all about the potential complications because, he realized, ignoring the risks helped him manage his fear.

Mary O'Donnell also turned her back on her concerns. But the feelings she conveyed in doing so were different from Douglass Cater's—ominously different. She entered the hospital without telling her children or her brother and sister. Lying on her side the afternoon before surgery, she stared vacantly at the blank wall beside her bed. In a shaky voice, she said that she was not afraid of surgery and that she had a positive attitude. Her only concern was that her physician be aware of her previous surgeries so he would handle her scars appropriately. She did not want to see the patient education film or think of the next day's events. She sounded terrified when she said, "I'm not ready to leave this world yet," and she drew the covers over her head.

The difference between Douglass Cater and Mary O'Donnell is the difference between healthy coping and unhealthy coping. When people like Mary O'Donnell withdraw prior to surgery, they may be signaling feelings of futility. Since the will to survive is essential to recovering well, such feelings can be catastrophic. Sadness, worry, nervousness, fear, and calm resolve are normal presurgical emotions which enable patients to work out their anxieties. When patients appear depressed and withdrawn, however, they may be signaling danger. Patients who are seriously depressed before surgery sometimes harbor death wishes, which they may not realize or want to admit. Nevertheless, they may view surgery as an easy avenue to death and thus be poor surgical candidates.

Andrew Razin, M.D., Ph.D., director of the Psychiatric Consultation-Liaison Service at North Central Bronx Hospital, Albert Einstein College of Medicine, warns of the dangers when seriously depressed patients go into surgery:

> There is considerable evidence to suggest that clinically depressed patients fare extremely poorly at cardiac surgery with a grossly excessive rate of mortality and of serious medical complications. Those who survive the postoperative course seem unlikely to benefit much from the surgery. Such patients should, whenever possible, have surgery postponed while treatment for the depression is instituted.

If you feel overwhelmed at the notion of surgery, if you find yourself dwelling on thoughts of death, if you have a history of depression, or if your family notices an abrupt change in your personality, the problem should be brought to your physician's attention.

Not all depression is portentous. In its least serious form, it is transient and lifts easily. Gordon Griffin experienced this kind of depression. He suddenly found himself feeling hopeless when he was told that his surgery had been preempted by an emergency.

"I was terrified of the prospect of surgery," he admitted. "In my experience, hospitals were places where people went to die, and I was mighty uncomfortable with the implications of lying in a hospital bed. I was even more distraught at the notion of being put to sleep. Someone else would have control over whether I lived or died! But I had to have the surgery, so I psyched myself up for it. I was into the countdown, and the morning of surgery, the nurse walks in and tells me my surgery had to be postponed for a day. You'd think I'd feel relieved because I had been granted a temporary stay of execution. Or angry because I had worked so hard to get myself ready and now I had to do it all over again. But I just went into this blue funk, which is not at all my style.

"After lunch, the social worker stopped in to see me. She said, 'Gee, you must really be angry.' I said, 'Angry? Why should I be angry? These things happen and it's no one's fault.' 'Well,' she said, 'If I had spent weeks preparing myself emotionally and then found out I had to do it again, I'd be absolutely furious. No one should have to do that. The prospect of heart surgery is tough enough without an additional emotional burden.'

"Yeah, it began to dawn on me. It wasn't fair. I began to feel this fury bubbling in my gut. First it kind of simmered. Then the bubbles boiled bigger, and I exploded. I was angry all day. I yelled at the nurse and I yelled at the intern and I yelled at the surgeon when he stopped by. But I didn't feel blue anymore."

Somewhat more intense was the depression Felix Amatta exhibited. When the nurse specialist visited Felix Amatta before his surgery, she sensed he felt hopeless and arranged for a psychiatric consultation. This man was not emotionally prepared for surgery, the psychiatrist agreed, but the psychiatrist felt that with a little more time, he would be able to manage it. The surgeon refused to operate until Felix Amatta was in a better frame of mind. He was discharged briefly, and when he felt ready, he rescheduled his surgery. The procedure was uneventful, and Felix Amatta recovered without serious complication.

George Coffer was also significantly depressed but his surgery could not wait. George Coffer, always tense, sad, and angry, tended to view life pessimistically. Becoming even more negative and distressed in the face of surgery, he appeared a poor surgical risk. However, a counselor, who spent time with him before and frequently after his operation, helped avert disaster. He suffered brief complications immediately after surgery and needed substantial encouragement to overcome his anxieties and become active. Because the counselor helped him face his fears, he made a complete recovery albeit with checkered progress. Over the ensuing months, George Coffer sought long-term counseling, which helped him cope with the difficulties of returning to work and maintaining his exercise program.

The experiences of George Coffer, Felix Amatta, and Mary O'Donnell occur infrequently. However, even the emotions which fall within the wide margins of normality can be difficult. Fortunately, about 10:00 the night before surgery, a nurse comes by with a sleeping pill. Although some patients worry about untoward reactions and refuse this sedative, every patient should take it. It is a blessed relaxant which draws a curtain over anxiety and permits a restful night's sleep.

## Points to Remember

❏ Take advantage of patient education classes and visits from professionals to ask all your questions.

❏ Keep pencil and paper handy for taking notes.

❏ Practice splinting the chest, techniques for getting out of bed, and lung exercises until you can do them without thinking.

❑ Try relaxation exercises and positive statements to help you manage difficult moments.

❑ If you or your family feels you are severely depressed before surgery, discuss the problem with your doctor.

## Chapter Four

# SURGERY AND THE ICU

The mind is a wondrous instrument that enables mothers to bear babies without pain-blocking drugs and soldiers to march into combat. The protective mechanism of the mind works effectively in the hours before surgery as well. To give it a boost, you will receive a sedative about an hour before you are wheeled from your room, and, incredible though it may seem, you will probably arrive in the operating room relaxed. Although some patients find this time frightening, they are the exception. Some patients feel so relaxed that they doze despite the bright lights and bustling activity around them. Others chat with the nurses and technicians as they perform their preoperative tasks. Thanks to the mind's protective mechanism and preoperative sedation, few patients remember these moments regardless of how alert they seem at the time.

## Preliminary Procedures in the Operating Room

Some patients would love it if they could be put to sleep before they were wheeled out of their rooms so they never had to see the operating room. Because of occasional unexpected delays and the axiom that patients should have as little anesthesia as possible, this is rarely done. You will be anesthetized in the operating room at some point during the preliminary procedures. Exactly when depends on the practices of each hospital, and these vary somewhat from one to another.

A number of procedures will take place before the actual surgery begins. Although slight variations are possible, these will include the following: You will be scrubbed from neck to foot with an orange-brown antiseptic called Betadine and covered with green sterile drapes. The team will affix EKG electrodes to your chest to monitor your heart and prepare several "lines" from which blood can be drawn, medications given, and vital processes monitored. Conventional intravenous tubes (IVs) will be placed in each arm to administer extra fluids. A slim plastic catheter will be inserted through the urethra into the bladder. The urine, which will drain through this catheter for the next couple of days, will be measured to evaluate kidney function and the possible need for additional fluids or medications. Another catheter will be fed into the main artery in the left wrist. Connected at the other end to a blood pressure monitor, this line will measure blood pressure in the arteries and provide an avenue from which to draw blood for analysis. Another line will be inserted near the collar bone into the subclavian vein in the neck and threaded through the heart into the artery leading to the lungs. By measuring the pressure in this artery, the anesthesiologist will be able to assess precisely how the heart is functioning. Near the end of surgery, two additional lines, chest tubes, will be inserted into the chest cavity through an incision in the skin beside the rib cage. These fat plastic tubes will permit residual blood and fluids to drain out of the chest after surgery and will remain in place for two days.

Admittedly, the image of a normally independent person immobile on an operating table serving as a human socket for various tubes is less than appealing. Yet, the procedures by which the catheters are affixed are not painful and the lines themselves provide the easiest avenue for giving medications and drawing specimens. More important, these lines permit exact evaluation of your physiological responses to the surgery and are therefore invaluable for your protection. In the first days after surgery, these tubes will be removed one by one. With the exception of removing the chest tubes, which can be momentarily painful, taking out the lines causes no discomfort. And each time one is removed, you can feel assured that you are making progress.

Either during or after the preliminary procedures, the anesthesiologist will slip some anesthesia into your IV, and you will fall into a deep, pain-free, sensation-free sleep. Unlike patients' experiences years ago, when now-antiquated anesthetic drugs were used, patients today are rarely aware that the anesthesia is taking effect. As one patient put it, "I was awake, and then I was awake again."

Once you are asleep, the anesthesiologist will insert one end of the endotracheal tube into your windpipe. The other end will be attached to a respirator, which will keep the lungs ventilated and permit the anesthesiologist to maintain an exact balance of gases during surgery. This endotracheal tube will still be in place when you wake up and will stay there for several hours or overnight, until the anesthetic has worn off sufficiently for you to breathe reliably and consistently. Next, the anesthesiologist may insert a tube through the nose and into the stomach to help prevent nausea after surgery. This too will be in place when you wake up.

## The Bypass Operation

The actual surgery begins when the skin is cut, the breast bone is split, and the rib cage is retracted. If the mammary artery is to be used, the surgeon prepares that artery next while another surgeon harvests the vein in one leg. Then, the thoracic surgeon carefully snips the pericardium, the protective sac which surrounds the heart. Once the heart is exposed, the surgeon prepares the circulatory system for detour through the heart-lung machine with the following four-step procedure: First, he creates an opening in the right atrium, the chamber of the heart which receives blood laden with waste products on its return trip from all parts of the body. Second, he makes a similar opening into the ascending aorta, the main artery which carries newly oxygenated blood throughout the body. Third, he injects heparin, a blood thinner, directly into the heart to prevent the blood from clotting while the heart-lung machine is in use. Last, he fits a tube into each of the two openings. When the other ends of these tubes are fitted into the heart-lung machine, the heart and lungs can be effectively detoured. Now, the blood can flow from the right atrium into the heart-lung machine, where waste products are removed and oxygen is replenished. Then the machine can pump the fresh blood back into the ascending aorta and from there throughout the body.

Once the heart-lung machine takes over the circulation, the heart is stopped and the blockages in the coronary arteries are bypassed using either a section of one of the large veins from the leg (usually the saphenous vein), the mammary artery inside the chest wall, or both. During the procedure, the surgeon usually bypasses all significantly blocked vessels unless they are too small or calcified, or unless the blocked arteries enter areas of the heart muscle which have been permanently scarred by previous heart attacks; restoring blood flow to such areas would be fruitless. On average, three or four arteries are bypassed, although surgeons occasionally do five or more when branches of the main arteries are individually obstructed.

To create each bypass made from the leg vein, the surgeon makes an opening in the aorta (the main artery carrying freshly oxygenated blood out of the heart) and another in the occluded artery below the blockage. By sewing one end of the bypassing vessel into the opening in the aorta and the other end into the opening in the coronary artery, the surgeon can reroute the flow of blood around the blockage. When the internal mammary artery is used, the surgeon snips this artery at a point on the chest wall just below the sternum, or breast bone. Leaving the artery attached at its origin, he creates a bypass by sewing the now-detached end into the coronary artery below the blockage. (See Appendix II.) This part of the procedure, when circulation is managed by the heart-lung machine, usually takes forty-five minutes to an hour.

The surgeon then checks the fit of the grafts. Once he is assured that the seal is perfect, he permits blood to flow along its new natural course and disconnects the heart-lung machine. At this point, the heart usually starts beating spontaneously, although it may need an electrical boost. Once it is beating, the blood thinner, which was injected into the heart to prevent clots while the blood circulated through the heart-lung machine, is counteracted with protamine, which the anesthesiologist injects. Just before closing the chest, the surgeon usually attaches a pair of fine wires to the heart. Protruding through the skin, these wires can be connected to an external pacemaker, which is sometimes necessary to regulate the heart for a few days. When this pacemaker is no longer needed, these wires are easily and painlessly removed.

## Waking from Anesthesia

Just as people in their own beds sometimes awake confused about what day it is or where they are, so patients often awake from anesthesia feeling bewildered. One patient recalled that as he awoke, he thought surgery hadn't started yet and wondered when it would begin. Then he heard his son shouting, seemingly from a great distance, "Your surgery is over and you're fine."

Another patient remembered total confusion. "I couldn't figure it out. Am I in surgery? Am I dead? Am I in the ICU? Then I heard someone mention Valium. That was a familiar term, so I figured I was alive, but I couldn't open my eyes. I struggled and struggled, but they wouldn't open  Then someone opened my eye and shined a light in it. I had a chance to see for a second, so I was sure

I was alive. I had a great sense of relaxation and well-being. I knew I was o.k."

Because it is so common to awake from general anesthesia feeling disoriented—after heart surgery or any other surgery—and because residual anesthesia makes people forgetful, the ICU nurses make a point of repeating the critical message: "Your surgery is over and you're fine."

"You're fine." That means that the electrocardiogram, which monitors the pace and rhythm of the heartbeat, shows that your newly repaired heart has tolerated being stopped, cooled, handled, fixed, rewarmed, and restarted. "You're fine" also means that the monitors which register blood pressure in the arteries and veins indicate that your blood is flowing properly and that the incisions are clotting effectively. It means that the blood samples which are periodically drawn and analyzed reveal that respiration is satisfactory. And it means that the urine output shows the kidneys functioning appropriately. Does it mean that you feel good? Probably not.

One patient described her first day after surgery this way: "I didn't have sharp pain. The drugs took care of that, and anyway, I've had abdominal surgery and, for me, the incision in the chest wasn't nearly as painful. I didn't hurt, but my chest felt like I had been hit by a Mack truck. My mouth was dry, and my body was soaked with sweat. I was so hot, and I couldn't move, and I couldn't get comfortable. And that damned breathing tube. That was the worst."

## Managing the Endotracheal Tube

The breathing tube, more than anything else, is a source of misery. In place for as little as a few hours of consciousness to as long as a day, it connects the pulmonary system to a respirator. During the early hours of consciousness, the respirator will breathe fully for you. As the after-effects of anesthesia wear off and you can begin

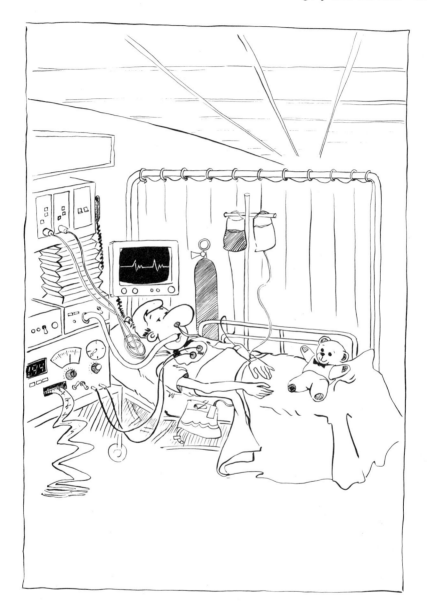

"Your surgery is over and you're fine."

to breathe independently, the respirator will provide intermittent support. And finally, when you can breathe reliably on your own, the tube will be removed.

Breathing with a respirator is difficult for most patients. As patients begin breathing independently, they frequently do not synchronize their breathing with the respirator. Instead of inhaling as the respirator pumps air into the lungs, they try to inhale as the respirator draws air out of the lungs. As patients experience this tug of war, they sense that they cannot get any air and they panic. This trouble occurs frequently, and although it is not serious, it can be frightening.

The nurses in the ICU are acutely sensitive to this difficulty and they are always on hand to coach patients and help them relax. If you encounter this problem, the nurse will probably tell you to stop breathing. If you stop trying to breathe on your own, you will stop fighting the machine and the sense of panic will disappear.

Under normal circumstances, after you stop breathing for a short while, you feel desperate for air. This feeling occurs when the blood needs oxygen. On the respirator, however, oxygen is fed to you continuously, so this feeling does not occur. You can successfully stop breathing, permit the respirator to do its job, and eliminate the sense of panic.

Conversely, once you are breathing independently enough so that the respirator provides only intermittent support, you may occasionally hear the respirator beep. This is not the signal of emergency. Rather, it is a reminder to breathe. The machine will guarantee that you get sufficient air. The nurses will be with you and will help you manage the respirator. While this is not a pleasant time, it is a safe time, and the nurses will help you get through it. Implementing relaxation techniques can be very helpful as well. So can repeating mantras of positive thoughts and concentrating on beautiful, sensuous images of another time and place.

Another difficulty with the respirator occurs during the moments when the intubation tube is cleared by suction, yet this procedure is vitally important. Before you can breathe deeply and perform your coughing exercises, suctioning is the only way to remove the secretions which formed in the lungs as a consequence of anesthesia. But the procedure puts pressure on the chest and makes you feel starved for air. Fortunately, the respiratory therapists are aware of the sensation and go out of their way to minimize it.

By the time you are first aspirated, you may feel comfortably secure with your respirator. Before your respiratory therapist can perform this maneuver, you must be taken off the respirator. This alone can be alarming. But before you can feel starved for air, the therapist will use a hand respirator to fill your lungs with air, and he will help you relax before continuing. To remove the mucus, the therapist will insert a slim (one-eighth inch in diameter) catheter through the intubation tube and withdraw the fluid. This is when the sensation of choking occurs. It is a normal sensation which lasts only eight to twelve seconds and is not dangerous. In between aspirations, the therapist will give you extra oxygen, and at no time will you be deprived of air. The entire procedure, including rests between suctionings, takes less than three minutes.

The last problem with the respirator occurs because the tube lies between the vocal cords, and while you are intubated you cannot talk. Again, the ICU nurses, who stay at the bedside almost continuously, are so experienced in the care of patients newly out of heart surgery that they can anticipate many of your thoughts, questions, and wishes. Nevertheless, not being able to communicate can be frustrating. One patient suffered because his lip was pinched between his intubation tube and his teeth, and he couldn't let the nurse know. Another patient awakened from surgery and felt frustrated because he couldn't ask all his questions about the operation. A third patient, so eager to convey his thoughts, tried scratching a message onto his nurse's arm.

Some former patients suggest a pencil and note pad to ease this frustration, but others feel that between the stupor of the drugs and the discomfort of having their arms strapped to IV boards, writing is difficult at best. Another patient recommends working up a list of questions and statements in advance and having a family member bring this into the ICU so you can simply point to your thoughts. You can also facilitate communication by working out your own brand of sign language with your family beforehand.

Ironically, patients occasionally worry about having the intubation tube removed. Some are concerned about discomfort from the procedure. However, with a cough from the patient and a gentle tug from the respiration therapist, the tube usually pops out without pain or other difficulty. Some patients also worry that they won't be able to breathe on their own. This fear, too, is unfounded.

"The last thing we want is to have to reintubate a patient," said Alan Stillerman, a respiratory therapist. "We can tell whether they're breathing efficiently by a simple blood test, and when we take a patient off the respirator, we know that patient is ready."

When the endotrachial tube is removed, patients are routinely put on supplemental oxygen to ease their breathing.

The best thing about being intubated is that it is over quickly. In one patient's words, "After that tube came out, I felt confident I would be o.k. I was so relieved to have survived to that point, I was just able to relax and let the nurses take care of me."

## Beginning the Work of Recovery

Although the breathing tube is usually out within twenty-four hours after surgery, some patients find the second postoperative day more difficult than the first. The anesthesia has worn off completely, and patients are more aware of their discomfort even though they are receiving pain medication. Moreover, while most patients would prefer to lie still and be left alone, they must begin the work of recovery. They must participate in their breathing treatments, turn from side to side, and sit up. These activities can be quite a chore at first. While they may be tiring and painful, they cannot—repeat: *cannot*—hurt the heart, dislodge the bypasses, or open the incision.

Martha Weinman Lear, who chronicled her husband's heart disease and surgery in a passionate narrative entitled *Heartsounds*, describes the discomfort her husband experienced as he dutifully tried to follow orders in the early days after his bypass operation:

> He had to cough to bring up mucus. That was imperative. If mucus were to block a bronchial tube, lung infections might develop.
>
> But in order to cough, he had to do what was diametrically opposed to instinct, which was to immobilize the chest. . . . One day a nurse suggested that he clutch a pillow tightly against his chest when he coughed, to help hold the chest wall together. [Editor's note: This is splinting, which was described in the preceding chapter.] That helped tremendously. He also discovered that if someone slapped his back, midway between the lungs, he could get up the mucus more easily.

And so we developed a routine: he would sit up, legs hanging over the edge of the bed, pillow clutched in his arms. "Okay, hit me," he would say. "Again—a little higher, a little to the left; there, *there, hit*," and at the moment I hit he would squeeze the pillow hard and cough and up would come, sometimes, a bit of mucoid matter—such a pathetic return for what it cost him, but a triumph nonetheless, a costly affirmation of life, health, restoration.

Once you are capable of taking deep breaths on your own, you will do your deep breathing exercises with the aid of a contrivance which measures your progress. These "incentive spirometers," as they are called, come in several varieties, and they require the kind of exercise you were taught before surgery: two deep breaths in through the nose and out through the mouth, and a third breath in followed by waiting for two seconds and coughing twice. If you cannot expand your lungs sufficiently on your own, you will begin with a device something like a manual respirator. This intermittent positive pressure breathing (IPPB) apparatus forces air into the lungs. Later, you will graduate to an incentive spirometer. Which appliance you start on is unimportant. What is important is that you expand your lungs and loosen the secretions so that pneumonia does not set in.

Also important is the notion that less than twenty-four hours after open chest surgery, you will be capable of performing these exercises and turning from side to side in bed. Once the intubation tube is out, you can sit on the edge of the bed, and one day later you will make your way to a chair. The power of the human body to heal itself is indeed remarkable.

## Disorientation in the ICU

Though intubation is uncomfortable and breathing and moving difficult, by far the most troubling aspect of the ICU is the disorientation which sometimes occurs.

Actually, it's a wonder that patients encounter as little disorientation as they do. Though modernization is slowly coming to intensive care units and some of the problems of ICUs are being solved, in most cases the very physical setup promotes disorientation. Most intensive care units are windowless wards, always light, always noisy. Ordinarily, these large, open rooms are lined with beds. Men and women lie separated from one another by only a curtain. Beside each bed is a full array of medical equipment—monitors, respirators, oxygen tanks, and IV trees which clank, rattle, beep, whirr, and whoosh. Periodically, a new patient is brought in after surgery, and occasionally a catastrophe occurs. Each of these events spurs additional commotion. In the middle of this arena sits the nurses' station, where telephones ring and where staff members hold conversations with little thought to keeping their voices hushed.

Into this chaos, where day is indistinguishable from night, patients emerge from heart surgery. The medications they receive enable them to drift in and out of sleep. However, these medications also make lights seem brighter and noises louder than they actually are. At the same time, these drugs lower people's tolerance for light and sound. Though patients are in a state of stress, they cannot release that stress as many people often do—by moving—and although they crave rest, rest in the ICU is next to impossible. Sleep deprivation aggravates the other problems, and disorientation can result, particularly among older patients. (Older patients may have atherosclerotic plaque in the arteries that lead to the head as well as in their coronary arteries. If plaque restricts the blood supply to the brain, the likelihood of confusion and disorientation increases.) Among all patients, nightmares are common, as are semi-awake hallucinations.

In the ICU, one patient saw huge black creatures whenever he closed his eyes. He recalled, "It was very surreal. I knew I was hallucinating, but that didn't make me feel any less terrified, and I strained to keep my eyes open. I couldn't close my eyes and rest until I was moved to my private room, and then—poof—I wasn't haunted anymore."

Once patients leave the ICU, these problems almost always vanish. Being in a more restful environment, where night is quiet and days are filled with recognizable structure, helps patients to reorient themselves. As they get out of bed and walk around, the circulation to their brains improves as well, and the monsters disappear.

In the early days of bypass surgery, severe mental disorders occurred frequently in the ICU. Today they are rare. Experts theorize that as the technology of bypass surgery improved and as patients grew to accept the surgery as commonplace, it became less traumatic. Yet temporary emotional upheaval seems more predominant among heart surgery patients than among other patients in the same environment. Tufts University professor of psychiatry Richard Blacher observed that among lung surgery, heart attack, and heart surgery patients assigned to the same ICU, severe difficulties were most likely among the heart surgery patients.

In the rare instances when psychosis in the ICU does occur, patients usually perceive their nurses as wanting to hurt them. This paranoia results from convoluted mental processes that work this way: Patients emerge from surgery feeling miserable and vulnerable. "Just turn out the lights, turn off the noises, and leave me alone," they wish. Contrary to these wishes, the nurses are forever turning them, suctioning them, and changing their IVs. Normally, this kind of treatment would enrage someone desperately wanting to be left alone. However, patients know that their lives depend on this care and they fear that if they become angry, the nurses will neglect them. So instead, they twist their anger and see it coming from nurses instead of from themselves. This unconscious mixup makes patients perceive their caretakers as hostile. Thus, a physician who became a patient in the very ICU where he had worked for years struck his nurse on the third day after his surgery!

Patients who worry that their nurses are out to hurt them usually realize that their perceptions are distorted, so they keep their thoughts secret. For years, some worry that they were crazy and that they will go crazy again. This fear is unfounded. Paranoia usually disappears permanently as soon as patients leave the ICU.

Despite the miasma of medication, patients are surprisingly alert once the anesthesia wears off, and they are often aware of what is going on around them even when they appear to be dozing. Unfortunately, sometimes they are alert enough to pick up fractions of conversations, but fuzzy enough to misinterpret what they hear or see. Thus, one patient misinterpreted the numbers on his blood pressure monitor and panicked that something dreadful was happening inside him.

"It's so important to air your fears," this patient advised. "If something doesn't look right or if you hear something frightening, call the nurse and ask. An explanation can be very reassuring."

## Complications in the ICU

Although being in the ICU is unpleasant, it is unquestionably the best place for patients newly out of surgery, for it is the ideal setup for catching complications. Opening the chest and manipulating the heart is, after all, major surgery. If superficial cuts or everyday hangnails can become infected, it should not be surprising that complications of various kinds can and do occur after surgery. For example, during the first eight to twelve hours, postoperative bleeding or the formation of blood clots sends a small percentage of patients back to the operating room. Usually this occurs before patients wake up from surgery, so they are rarely aware of the complication until it is history. And, while the incident can frighten the family, surgery is the quickest and safest way to solve the problem.

Other potential problems include imbalanced electrolytes, wound infections, fevers, and irregular heartbeats. As a consequence of surgery, the electrical system which regulates the heartbeat can be disrupted, causing the heart to beat too slowly, too quickly, or unevenly. These palpitations can be frightening when they suddenly make your EKG monitor beep or create the feeling that horses are galloping in your chest. But palpitations are easily and quickly corrected. In addition, particularly among patients whose hearts were pumping inefficiently before surgery, extra fluids may build up in the lungs and elsewhere in the body.

A patient who had this problem laughed as she told this story: "The doctor had just finished examining me and turned to the nurse and said, 'She's in failure.' Oh, my God, I thought, I'm dying. I just lay there and thought about my life and my grandchildren and I wondered if I'd ever see them again. The nurse must have noticed something was wrong, because she asked me. I said, 'I heard the doctor say I was in failure.' So the nurse said—she was smart—'Mrs. Melatta, do you know what that means? Failure is short for congestive heart failure and it just means that your body is retaining too much fluid. It's probably from the extra fluids you got during surgery. We'll give you a diuretic to take care of it.' Sure enough, I was fine, but it's so easy to get scared."

On rare occasion, heart attacks, strokes, perforated ulcers, and kidney failure occur. Patients with diabetes are especially vulnerable to kidney failure. Mild heart attacks immediately before, during, or after surgery occur in 2% to 4% of cases and often do not delay recovery. The risk of serious heart attack is less than 1%. Strokes are similarly rare in younger patients, but become a major concern with patients older than seventy-five. In earlier years, when the technology surrounding the surgery and use of the heart-lung machine were relatively primitive, these complications were more prevalent, and, as Martha Weinman Lear's book *Heartsounds* conveys, they are tragic. Today, however, permanent neurological problems are rare.

When complications such as strokes or kidney failure involve body systems outside the expertise of the cardiologist or surgeon, these doctors frequently consult with an internist who specializes in the area of the patient's problem. Similarly, cardiologists sometimes consult with their colleagues if a patient has a particularly menacing arrhythmia or other cardiac complication. These consultants, as well as the team approach to patient management, assure the best and most comprehensive patient care. If you or a member of your family feels that your complications are excessive or that your progress is unreasonably slow, feel free to ask your doctors for a consultation with another expert. Most physicians do not take offense at such requests. In fact, they often welcome the opportunity to confer with a respected colleague. A consultant may shed valuable light on your difficulties. At the very least, another opinion may confirm your physician's views and thereby help to assuage your worries.

Complications, serious or slight, understandably cause anguish and fear. When they occur, it often helps to be creative in managing them. Thus, the wife of a patient whose short-term memory disappeared for about three weeks helped her husband cope with the problem by bringing him a pad and pencil and encouraging him to keep notes. It also helps to remember the statistics: 25% of bypass patients encounter some kind of setback. While the likelihood of complication varies with each patient's age and unique medical profile, as many as 99.5% of patients recover without serious complications.

In part, the risks are so low because they are spotted and treated swiftly. This is the value of the intensive care unit. Here, computers register vital body processes and keep medications properly controlled. Every emergency and diagnostic tool is immediately available. And specially trained professionals provide expert care and constant attention.

"Thank God for those nurses," extolled an eighty-five-year-old man who, because of several postoperative set-backs, spent more than a week in the ICU. "My Annie, she was an angel. She knew just how to fix the pillow under my knees. She would wipe my head with a cold cloth. I'm a foolish old man, I guess, but in those gentle hands I felt love."

Older patients tend to recover more slowly than younger patients, and those with damaged heart muscles usually have more difficulty than those whose hearts are healthy, but almost everyone improves. One sixty-five-year-old patient illustrated this miracle of recovery. He had emergency bypass surgery after a serious heart attack. In the ICU he was disoriented for three days. His heart rhythm and blood pressure took nearly a week to stabilize, and throughout that time his cardiologist worried that he might die. Although most patients stay in the ICU no more than three days, this patient could not be moved for eight. Finally, he was able to leave the ICU, and two days after that, he greeted guests in the solarium at the end of the hall.

Ironically, even in the ICU, progress occasionally brings difficulties of its own. As patients become more alert and less preoccupied with pain, they sometimes become aware of new and troubling emotions. A few, though they are aware that their surgery was life-saving, grieve for their bodies, which they perceive as mutilated, and even some strong men may become tearful. Some patients, particularly those who crave control over their lives, feel frustrated by their helplessness and dependency on machines and medical personnel.

A middle-aged woman experienced this fury the third day after surgery. "I was sitting up in bed breathing this cold dry air [supplemental oxygen] and just feeling furious. My husband asked me why I was so angry, and I told him I felt frustrated because I was powerless. He knows me so well. He patted my hand and gave me a terrific suggestion. 'You're so intent on having control,' he said. 'Why don't you just decide to exercise your control over yourself?' So I did. I really worked at being cooperative. It was a good plan for me."

The last day or so in the ICU, patients often discover they can't remember the hours immediately before and after surgery. This amnesia is a normal function of the mind's protective mechanism. If you encounter this problem and find it distressing, ask your nurse or your family to help you reconstruct the missing hours.

You may also be surprised to discover you have gained weight, even though you have been eating next to nothing. These pounds represent the excessive fluids that you received during surgery and will disappear before you are discharged.

Discomfiting though these problems are, you will not become aware of them until you begin to feel better, so in their own way, they are a sign of progress. Next step: a regular room.

## Points to Remember

❏ You will probably feel calm going into surgery and will not be aware of being put to sleep.

❑ In ICU, do your best to relax and permit the nurses to take care of you.

❑ Try not to fight the respirator.

❑ If you see or hear anything that worries you, ask your nurse about it.

❑ Disorientation, amnesia, and weight gain are normal.

Chapter Five

# STEP-DOWN CARE

"Praised be the moment they wheeled me out of that intensive care unit. I just knew the worst was over," one patient exclaimed.

Most people greet this move with joy. A regular hospital room signifies medical progress and promises rest. Yet a regular room can feel disconcertingly strange to those who have grown accustomed to ICU routine. Patients who found the constant attention of medical personnel comforting sometimes worry that, once in a regular room, their problems will go unnoticed. Sometimes just the change in surroundings, personnel, and routines feels threatening.

Under any circumstances, moving from a familiar environment to an unfamiliar one causes stress. When people have been ill, all their vulnerabilities are exaggerated, and their vulnerability to moves from one hospital setting to another is no exception. Patients recovering from heart attacks, for example, sometimes encounter difficulties attributed to stress when they are abruptly transferred from the coronary care unit to a regular hospital room. However, if patients are told about the transfer in advance and if they are moved by people they know, they manage it more easily.

These findings translate neatly for heart surgery patients leaving the ICU. Ideally, hospital personnel whom you know—a counselor, nurse, patient education specialist, aide, or orderly—will accompany you during the move or visit soon after. Perhaps you can arrange for your spouse or children to be present. At the very least, take the opportunity to ask about your new home. The most important question is this: "How, in this less intensively supervised environment, will anyone know if I am in trouble?"

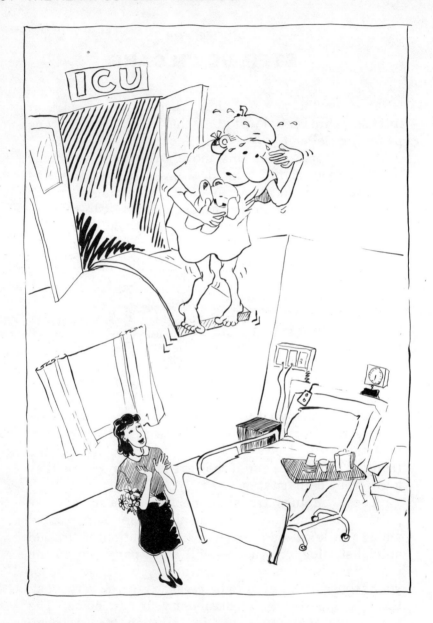

Under any circumstances, moving from a familiar environment to an unfamiliar one causes stress.

# Telemetry

Any hospital with a good coronary care program reduces the supervision of its bypass patients gradually. Patients leaving the ICU move to a room where each patient's heart continues to be monitored. In many hospitals these rooms form a separate "telemetry" unit. In some hospitals, they are scattered within a general medical-surgical unit. Regardless of the setup, for their first several days out of ICU, patients continue to have their heart rhythms monitored either by a bedside EKG or by a beeper-like device which they wear and which records every heartbeat on a television monitor at the nurses' station. This monitoring is so scrupulous that often, when an irregular heartbeat occurs, doctors and nurses are attending to it before the patient realizes what has happened.

During the first days out of the ICU, nurses are never far away. Patients don't even get out of bed without a nurse standing by. Little by little, the nurses lengthen their tether, and by the time the heart monitor is removed, patients have had ample time to gain confidence in themselves and their newly repaired hearts. From the first hour in the telemetry unit, however, the theme is independence. Hospital personnel think of patients not as sick but as recovering from surgery. This recovery demands that patients assume responsibility for taking care of themselves.

"We discourage private duty nurses," said Barbara Friedman. "If patients are going to leave this hospital to lead normal lives, they've got to see themselves as independent. We didn't operate on them so someone else could take care of them."

## Reestablishing Independence

Predictably, patients respond differently to this firm attitude. Those who relish taking control of their lives often embrace every facet of this responsibility in an attempt to minimize the passivity that hospital routine imposes on them. With the go-ahead from their nurses, they devise a strict schedule for walking, resting, and practicing breathing exercises. They monitor their reactions closely and report any concerns to their caretakers.

While all the possibilities may not be immediately apparent, there are, in fact, several ways in which you can take charge. Responsibility begins with accepting the commitment to work in the face of discomfort: trying to stand up straight even when your chest incision seems to pull your shoulders down; walking without a limp even if your leg incision begs to be coddled; breathing deeply when it feels as though another cubic centimeter of air simply won't fit.

"I was determined to follow orders to exercise," one patient acknowledged. "I said I was doing it for my family, and I have no doubt that their encouragement was part of my motivation. But secretly, I did it for myself. Setting a goal and striving to meet it . . . how can I explain it? It was a challenge. It was a triumph. It was like beating my own record in the fifty-yard dash."

You can also take charge of your medications. You can monitor your pain killers, for example. Once you are out of intensive care, your pain medication will be prescribed according to your weight and the estimated time for medication to take effect. However, physicians tend to undermedicate. Moreover, when physicians order doses to be repeated every four to six hours, nurses often deliver the drugs closer to the six-hour interval. As a result, you may encounter more pain than you need to.

Pain is demoralizing and exhausting. Worse, it keeps you from resting thoroughly and exercising vigorously. If you are to work at recovering effectively, you need your pain medication frequently enough to prevent intense pain.

There is a difference between pain and discomfort. Discomfort implies an unpleasant awareness. It is mild enough that it remains in the background, but it is definitely present. Pain, in contrast, screams for attention. It prevents reading, moving, even listening to conversation. When pain medication fails to reduce pain to discomfort, you must tell your nurse, who can often juggle the dosage and scheduling of the drugs. These medicines work best when the blood level of the drug stays constant; once the blood level falls off and pain builds up, you will need more medication to get relief. Thus, adjusting the interval at which the medication is given can make a significant difference in its effectiveness and, in the long run, reduce the quantity of medicine you take.

In addition, it's a good idea, if you can, to take pain medication forty-five minutes to an hour before doing physical therapy or respiration exercises. This timing assures that the medication is delivering the maximum relief when you need it most. These are all factors which you can monitor.

When problems occur and your nurse cannot solve them, it is important to discuss them with the physician in charge. In the unlikely circumstance that the physician fails to respond as well, you can turn to whomever your hospital designates as the patients' advocate. Personnel structures vary from hospital to hospital, but in any good hospital you should be able to identify someone who will speak on your behalf. Perhaps it is a nurse supervisor, a patient education specialist, a clinical nurse specialist, or a social worker. Hopefully, by the time problems of this nature erupt, you and your family are well enough attuned to the hospital hierarchy that you or someone close to you can identify the appropriate resource.

As for other medications, you must know about each drug you take—what it is, what it does, and what its potential dangers are. This is an ideal time to pay attention to that information.

Constipation, an unpleasant side effect of pain medication and the sedentary nature of recovery, is another area where you can take charge.

"Make sure you're getting a stool softener," advises a nurse-turned-patient. "Drink lots of water, unless you are having problems with water retention. And make a concerted effort to eat vegetables, fruits, salads, and fiber cereals."

While some patients seek every opportunity for responsibility, other patients prefer to relinquish their care to others. Patients who embrace a passive role sometimes find it difficult to overcome inertia. Such was the case with James Nicholson. At sixty-one, he had a ten-year history of chest pain. His father had died of heart disease at age forty-six, and his brother had had a severe heart attack three years earlier. James Nicholson's angina, which steadily got worse until he had surgery, together with his family history convinced him that he was next. Although surgery quieted his angina, James Nicholson had trouble overcoming his fears. Once out of ICU, he was afraid to challenge himself. He quickly—too quickly—gave in to weakness and fatigue. He complained that even modest physical therapy exercises drained his energy. Worse, he dreaded leaving the hospital and was not eager to hurry his progress along.

Patients like James Nicholson, who have been conditioned to fear exertion by years of pain, often resist testing their surgery, especially if they worry that their discomforts suggest continuing heart disease. If you are disinclined to work at recovery, you must find a way to overcome your resistance. Since the heart is a muscle and muscles thrive on exercise, you must participate in your recovery exercises or you will not benefit from your surgery. If you avoid exercising because you are frightened by sensations in your chest, you must learn more about what you are feeling.

Everyone has pain at the incision site, which is reduced to discomfort by medication. When you first wake up from anesthesia, you will be aware of this pain as well as the pain from your leg incision. By the third or fourth day, your pain should be reduced to a mild annoyance and should be controllable by pills rather than injections. The various healing pains which you experience do not worry your doctor, and they shouldn't worry you.

Some patients say with assurance that healing pains are distinctly different from angina. Angina responds to nitroglycerine; healing pains do not. While angina tends to come with exertion in general, pain from incisions and muscles strained during surgery is more likely to be associated with specific movements, even breathing.

Admittedly, these descriptions are less than definitive. Pain is highly subjective and personal, and when people are concerned about their health, they can become confused about their perceptions. Do not worry in silence. If you are confused about how to interpret your pain, discuss it with your doctor, nurse, or physical therapist. Nurses and physical therapists see hundreds of patients recovering from heart surgery and they are in a particularly good position to evaluate your pain. Ask them if they think your pain is unusual, and try to describe what you feel. Is the sensation sharp or dull? Does it feel like a squeeze, a stab, a stick, or a weight? Is it intermittent or sustained? What causes it? Does it occur at a predictable time of day or night? What other sensations come at the same time? What relieves the pain? The more specifically you can describe your pain, the more accurately the professionals can diagnose its cause. If you are convinced that your pain is not dangerous, you will have an easier time persevering, and persevere you must.

Getting well is a lot of work.

# The Nature of Recovery

Even patients who embrace the work of recovery, however, feel tentative and uncertain. "Was my surgery a success?" nearly everyone wonders. "Will I be able to walk to the bathroom? Play golf? Return to work? Make love?" These concerns are natural, particularly since recovery is not characterized by steady improvement. All patients have good days, when a sense of progress and well-being prevail, and bad days. Aches and pains, fatigue, weakness, and other minor setbacks happen routinely, and when they occur, worry and frustration often follow.

"I think we tend to jump to conclusions too quickly," a patient observed. "The minute I felt good, I expected I'd always feel good. Then, when I felt less good, I was sure something terrible had happened."

Most patients are unusually alert to their bodies now. They measure every inch of new-found strength and worry that every twinge might signal a setback. Another patient observed that insecurity breeds apprehension. A physician himself, he recalled being obsessed about a sensation in his chest which he couldn't identify. "During surgery, the attachments of my heart were somehow disturbed, and my heart was more mobile in my chest than it had been. Lying on my left side at night, it felt as though my lung was being compressed with each heartbeat. I worried about that until I realized what it was."

# Anger

Harbored fears erode the temperament, and when patients are worried—consciously or unconsciously— they sometimes become uncharacteristically irritable. Paul Stevens, for example, became argumentative and stubborn shortly after he was moved out of ICU. Always reasonable and cooperative before, he now refused to take his medicine or even look at his tray at mealtime.

"There was one nurse who dropped by every afternoon just to talk," this patient revealed months after his surgery. "She could sense when patients were upset. She'd come in and sit down on the edge of the bed as though there weren't anything else to do in the world. She asked about my wife, and I told her the whole story. It was a second marriage for both of us. We were married just a year when I had my surgery. Laura was working and visiting me and trying to do everything around the house. And of course, she was worried. As I told this nurse all about my wife, I began to realize that I was scared for Laura, and scared for myself, and scared for us. Talking to her helped me to gain a new perspective on my anger."

Anger is a common emotion in the days and weeks after surgery. To observers it often seems unwarranted, and it is often misdirected at the people the patients love most. Sometimes, it is disguised fear, but not always. It can stem from the frustration that patients experience when they tackle the tasks of recovery diligently and feel their bodies aren't responding quickly enough. And sometimes it grows out of a sense of impotence which comes from lying in a hospital bed.

The best antidote to all these emotions is talk. When people address their problems, they take the first important step to resolving them. Fortunately, under the stresses of this hospital experience, emotional controls loosen, and many people can reach a level of candor they never had before.

For example, Diane Murray was able to address the denial she clung to before her surgery and resolve her anxieties. "I couldn't admit that I was worried before the surgery," she acknowledged some weeks after her discharge from the hospital. "It was as though if I admitted I was scared, something terrible would happen, and as long as I kept a stiff upper lip, everything would be fine.

Afterwards, though, the reality hit. Now, I can accept that I have heart disease. I can accept my mortality. And I can concentrate on exercising, eating right, and prolonging my life."

For Tony Mendoza, the biggest problem was feeling like a child. "It's bad enough you have to exercise when they tell you and take your medicine when they tell you. But you can't even eat when you want to. They bring you this trash somebody calls food, and expect you to eat it whether you're hungry or not," he complained to the nursing supervisor.

"You'd rather have some nice lasagna at a candlelit table for two?" she suggested.

The next evening, Tony Mendoza sat down to dinner at 7:00, the time he usually ate dinner at home. With the nursing supervisor's encouragement and assistance, Elizabeth Mendoza made her husband's favorite dish, which she reheated in the microwave oven in the nurses' lounge. It wasn't quite the same as dinner at home, but it helped to reassure Tony Mendoza that he was a man who had the power to make a decision.

Despite the frustrations, the recuperative powers of the body carry on. Just four or five days after surgery, most patients—even men and women well on in years—look healthy. They can cough, breathe deeply, and do their physical therapy exercises without apparent distress. Wearing bathrobes and slippers, these patients stand casually in the hall chatting with each other and their visitors. Even they are amazed at the speed of their progress.

Yet this well-being is a fragile thing, as one patient's experience dramatizes.

"I was feeling great," fifty-year-old Marvin Dolan recalled. "It was less than one week after surgery, and I really was doing very well. I had had a lot of company. We talked and joked, and when they left, I walked them down the hall. I didn't realize it at the time, but I had overdone it. The next day, I had no steam at all. It took a few days before I regained the ground I had lost."

Marvin Dolan's tenuous perch between growing strength and impending setback is typical. As patients inch forward, they often become unusually contemplative. It's common for bypass patients to reevaluate their philosophies and priorities. Many ponder the possibilities of changing to less stressful jobs, retiring early, spending more time with their families. Even hard-nosed business people frequently turn nostalgic and sentimental. As one Wall Street lawyer coined metaphors about red and yellow leaves dancing outside his window, he sounded more like William Wordsworth than A. Steven Danforth III.

Steven Danforth, never sentimental, was suddenly wistful about autumn landscapes. Diane Murray, who had never acknowledged feeling anything but fine, was admitting she had been too afraid to face her fears. Mild-mannered Paul Stevens turned ugly and irascible in the days after his surgery. People who have always prided themselves on their stoicism dissolve into tears without apparent provocation, and understandably, they worry they have permanently lost their self-control. Such changes in temperament, especially when they are characterized by upwelling emotions, occur frequently as patients settle into the second stage of recovery. These changes are temporary and usually vanish within a couple of months.

# Depression

On the fourth or fifth day (perhaps sooner and perhaps not until weeks later), many patients encounter depression, sometimes for the first time in their lives. For some, the depression amounts to no more than fleeting blue moments. Others experience a dense fog of hopelessness and despair.

"It's a rare patient who experiences no reactive depression whatsoever," said counselor Sally Kolitz. "But these feelings are normal and self-limiting. Painful and frightening though they may be, they are not serious."

Amy Foster recalled the moment depression hit her, on the fifth day after her surgery. "I was standing over the sink in the bathroom washing my hair, and I started to cry. I didn't feel particularly sad or worried, but I couldn't help myself. I just sobbed my heart out. Oh, what was happening to me?"

Diane Murray said her depression set in when she suddenly became convinced she would never recover. "I was so elated when they told me I could leave the ICU. I was out of there just two days after surgery and I thought, boy, I'm going to set a record here. After I was in my room for about an hour, the nurse came in to help me get into a chair and moving was tougher than in the ICU. My chest incision hurt more, and I felt so weak I thought I would sink right through the chair. I was devastated."

"You bet I feel blue," said Michael Conran, a thirty-five-year-old insurance agent who had emergency surgery while he was on a business trip two thousand miles from home. "I just got a new job, and I'm wondering if I'm gonna keep it. I live to play baseball, and I'm not sure I'm ever gonna swing a bat again. Not this season, that's for sure. I've just spent six months building up my body in the gym, and now I'm gonna lie here and watch it go soft."

Another patient echoed this young man's concerns when, on his fifth postoperative day, he worried if he would ever ski again or whether he would always feel deprived because he couldn't eat his favorite chocolate cake.

Patients whose very survival lifted them into euphoria sometimes claim they never felt true depression. The subdued feelings they called depression were nothing more than subsiding ecstasy. For others, feelings of hopelessness weigh heavily. Regardless of degree, these emotions and the tears that frequently accompany them are a natural response to an overload of emotional and physical stresses. After all, every patient who reaches this point has, within the recent past, confronted his mortality, surrendered to the manipulation of his body, trusted his very breath to people he barely knows, and returned to consciousness in the cacophony of the ICU.

All patients are weakened by the operation and the anemia that normally follows it. Many become exhausted in the ICU, where they find sleeping difficult. To make matters worse, they receive pain medication which triggers depression as a side effect. Is it any wonder that the mind rebels? Controls are loosened as the mind takes time out to heal itself. Anger, poor concentration, memory loss, difficulty reading and thinking of words, and seemingly unprovoked weepiness occur when the mind steps off guard. Blue feelings and tears can descend spontaneously on and off for up to three months. Gradually, they recede. And then, for most patients, they disappear.

To ease depression, be realistic in your expectations. Since heart surgery causes major physical and emotional disruption, healing takes a long time. Gains are tangible, but they are sometimes small, sometimes halting. Even after patients are home, the gains play tug of war with weakness and fatigue. When fatigue sets in, everything hurts more and emotions are more difficult to manage. Gradually the good days win out. But although patients can resume most of their activities within six weeks, many admit it takes months, some say a year, before they feel like themselves in all respects. Consequently, you will do yourself a favor if you expect the pace of recovery to be slow and uneven. Conversely, if you are impatient with yourself and unrealistic in your short-term goals, you will set the stage for depression.

In addition to having realistic expectations, you can benefit from accepting depression and other temporary personality changes with equanimity. If you understand that these emotional shifts are normal and temporary, you will work through them more quickly than if you harbor fears that surgery mutilated your mind.

During this period when emotional controls are loosened, patients who had unusually frightening experiences years before occasionally dredge them up. One patient, for example, relived his childhood horrors as a prisoner in Auschwitz. Although he had successfully coped with these memories for more than fifty years, during the week after surgery he began to be plagued with nightmares so terrifying that he contemplated suicide. Occurrences like this are rare and usually temporary. They are best managed by talking them through, preferably in consultation with a professional counselor.

Although emotional distress is troublesome, you and your loved ones should not find it threatening, provided you see two things: one, that it lifts from time to time; and two, that it is not so oppressive that it keeps you from the activities that promote recovery. When depression becomes deeply entrenched, patients stop caring about whether they develop pneumonia or circulatory problems. When they stop caring, they stop doing their deep breathing and physical therapy exercises, and they fail to progress.

With the physical aspects of recovery, as with depression, patients' experiences vary. Many have no difficulty coughing or breathing deeply after the third or fourth day. Yet others complain that the respiration therapy is the most agonizing part. Some patients complain about their incisions when they walk and about a general numbness in their chests. Other patients are bothered most by shoulder and back muscle strain, a result of the rib cage being retracted during surgery. Still other patients say they never feel unbearable pain but find they are periodically overcome by weakness and exhaustion. Others worry about their inability to concentrate and gaps in their memory—both normal products of stress, anesthesia, and medication.

During this phase of recovery, do not be surprised if you feel nauseated and find food distasteful. Anesthesia, medications, and electrolyte disturbances can all contribute to this problem. Eating well promotes healing, however, and on the basis of this rationale you may indulge in your most tempting favorites, even a corned beef sandwich or chile con carne.

Clinical nurse specialist Barbara Friedman advises, "During recovery, the body needs a full range of nutrients to repair itself. At this point, it's much more important for patients to eat well than follow a diet plan. If they would enjoy a rare steak and french fried potatoes, bring them in. When patients eat the foods they enjoy, they get a psychological lift, too. When their appetite returns in a week or two, that's the time to get serious about lowering fats and cholesterol."

Winking, she added, "It makes the families feel awfully good when they can bring in food. It's great when they can make a positive contribution to the recovery of the person they love."

## Medical Complications

No matter how dedicated patients are to promoting their recovery, complications occasionally thwart the progress. As a rule, older and sicker patients encounter more difficulties than younger, more vigorous patients. Patients with atherosclerosis of the arteries that feed the head often suffer from tiny clots in their brains. These can cause neurological symptoms and can affect word recall and memory sometimes for months.

Smokers, like people with asthma, chronic bronchitis, and other lung diseases, are bound to have more trouble than nonsmokers. During the early postoperative hours, when patients are intubated, smokers need to be suctioned more frequently than nonsmokers. They find the breathing and coughing exercises more painful, and they recover more slowly.

As one patient who had been on oxygen for eight days after his surgery put it, "I smoked for years. Now I'm paying for it."

Whether patients smoke or not, they occasionally confront wound infections, systemic infections, clots in the lungs, and an inflammation in the chest called postcardiotomy syndrome, which causes fever, other flu-like symptoms, and depression. Some 40 to 50% of patients experience abnormal heartbeats. Although these arrhythmias can be severe, they are usually not serious. Understandably, however, they can be distressing, especially when they occur after patients have been taken off their telemetry monitors and then have to be reattached.

"In this business, every step is a mark of progress or regression," one cardiologist and former patient explained. "In the ICU, every time they take out a line, you think, aha, I'm moving along. Then you leave the ICU—more progress. Then you can get out of bed unsupervised. Then they take you off the monitor, and you figure you're almost home. Then you fibrillate and you're back on the monitor. I'm a physician. I should know better. But when it happened to me, I really got bummed out. I was convinced I'd never get better."

He did, of course. Most patients do. One of our patients, sixty-eight years old, suffered from such severe angina that he could barely walk before his surgery. When he entered the hospital, his blood pressure was so low he was nearly dead. He was in ICU eight days, and had a dreadful time with postoperative psychosis. After seventeen days in the hospital, he went home and was fine.

Another patient, sixty years old, should have had an easy time because, except for his clogged arteries, he was healthy and vigorous. But eight days into recovery, he developed a wound infection and clots in his lungs. Although he stayed in the hospital nearly three weeks, he left expecting an uncompromised recovery.

Almost always, complications are more distressing than they are serious. And almost always they can be corrected.

# Resolving Concerns

Throughout the recovery process, but especially when unexpected concerns arise, patients and their families yearn for explanations and reassurance from their surgeons. Sometimes, surgeons offer veritable panaceas in their daily visits. They listen to their patients' hearts and comment on what they hear. They sit down, answer all their patients' questions, and ask questions of their own, indicating that they are aware of and concerned about each patient's unique circumstances. All too often, however, the surgeons remain maddeningly out of reach. At worst, they don't visit and they don't return phone calls. More commonly, they are present, but distant and aloof. Even when they visit daily, they frequently hang on to the door post as if to say, "Don't expect a lengthy conference." When patients yearn to tackle their list of questions and sense their physician's impatience, their frustration and fear can intensify.

You need not endure this frustration passively. Certainly the surgeon is an ideal person to answer questions, and if you wish to consult your physician, try to make an appointment to do so. Sometimes, physicians remain distant for fear that, given the chance, their patients will trap them in endless conversation. To counter that worry, you might approach your physician saying, "I have five questions I'd like to ask you," or "I need fifteen minutes to talk to you. Could you please arrange that for tomorrow?"

It's natural to feel that since the surgeon fixed the heart, he's the best person to answer questions about it. But this presumption isn't necessarily so, especially for surgeons who are better at operating than communicating. On the other hand, many nurses are knowledgeable professionals trained to educate patients. A patient educator or clinical nurse specialist can probably provide thorough, satisfying answers. So can your cardiologist, other physicians, physician's assistants, and the therapists who work with heart patients regularly.

Occasionally, patients openly express their fury at the unavailability of their physicians. Confrontation can be unpleasant, but patients who draw battle lines because their physicians won't satisfy their need to talk are conquering the bigger struggle. They are feeling well enough that they can concentrate on something other than their survival. How refreshing to be able to solve problems like these!

During this second stage of recovery, we found that patients' concerns tend to follow a predictable course. At first, they worry about setbacks, later about dependency. Ultimately, most patients grow strong enough and feel so good that they have nothing serious to worry about anymore. For some, there is the lingering concern about having the staples or stitches in their chests removed. However, once this minor procedure is over, patients who had worried about it invariably respond, "Is that all? Oh, my goodness!"

With the staples or stitches out, there is little to keep patients in the hospital any longer. It's time for discharge instructions and the long-awaited trip home.

# Points to Remember

❑ Do your lung and physical exercises religiously, if possible, about an hour after taking pain medication.

❑ Talk to your nurse or doctor if your pain is not kept at a tolerable level of discomfort.

❑ Prevent constipation by taking a stool softener; drinking water; and eating fruits, vegetables, and whole grains.

❑ Accept anger and depression as normal consequences of weakness, surgery, and stress. Be prepared for good days and bad days.

❏ Try to keep realistic expectations for recovery.

❏ If you feel frustrated because you cannot talk to your surgeon at length, arrange to take up your concerns with another professional.

## Chapter Six

# RECOVERING AT HOME

Going home—hallelujah! In anticipation of the great day, there's much to learn: what medications you need; how these new medications affect other medications you take from time to time—aspirin for headaches, antihistamines for allergies, and antacids for indigestion, for example; what you can eat; how you will spend your days; what kind of exercise you can do; what you can't do; when you can travel, go back to work, make love.

As you prepare to cut the umbilical cord of the hospital, there is so much information to assimilate that many hospitals offer discharge classes. In other hospitals, patients receive the information via closed circuit television, booklets, or chats with the patient educator. Regardless of how the information is proffered, patients characteristically feel overwhelmed by a cascade of details they fear they will never remember. That's normal. Take notes. Invite the family to sit in. Ask questions. Repeat the questions. There are too many details for anyone to recall. What's more, just as the stress of the preoperative hours interfered with concentrating and remembering, so the excitement and concerns at the time of discharge shorten the memory and make paying attention difficult. Sensitive nurses, therapists, and physicians realize that you cannot absorb all this information at once, and they are prepared to repeat themselves.

## The Theme of Recovery

Regardless of how discharge information is presented, these underlying messages should come through:

Recovery is not yet completed even though discharge from the hospital means that it is well underway. For at least the next six weeks—and maybe for as long as several months—you must remain dedicated to the hard work of recovery. Inherent in those duties are respecting the healing process with its associated discomforts and fatigue, being dedicated to a lifestyle governed by exercise and rest, and accepting the emotional trials which are characteristic of this arduous recuperation.

Patients often go home before all complications— infections and irregular heartbeats, for example— are resolved. Despite continuing difficulties, the very fact that you are being discharged means that the complications are not worrisome and can be managed safely from home.

Although you may have spent many years plagued by angina, you are not a cardiac cripple now. You put up with all the difficulties and discomforts associated with surgery because surgery held the promise for a higher quality of life. Getting on with that life should be your first priority and continuing the work of recovery your immediate goal.

All patients go home with questions and uncertainties. Understandably, some even fear going home. While they were in the hospital, they could count on skilled professionals to manage any setbacks. Surely, every patient who experienced a sudden arrhythmia which brought the nurses scurrying wonders, "What if it happens at home?"

Because patients routinely go home with unsettling discomforts, many good hospitals and surgeons encourage patients to call a knowledgeable liaison—perhaps a patient educator, a counselor, or an information specialist in the surgeon's office—when concerns arise during the first week at home.

"Our patients go home knowing we welcome their calls," said clinical nurse specialist Barbara Friedman. "Usually they call with specific questions, but sometimes they call just to talk. One patient called after he had been home a week to say, 'I had heart surgery and I just realized its significance.'"

This kind of liaison provides security and buffers the transition between hospital and home, especially when patients feel apprehensive because they cannot interpret their discomfort. You must not hesitate to contact this person if you have worries or questions. Resist the inclination to ignore your concerns out of consideration for a medical professional's busy day. Gnawing insecurity can warp your self-confidence. In contrast, if you resolve your concerns and questions, you will gain confidence and your concerns will diminish. Within a week or so, you will probably feel secure enough that the frequency of your calls will fall off.

Many patients report that their first week at home was more difficult than their last days in the hospital. Going home can emphasize patients' weakness and vulnerability, just as moving from the ICU to a regular room had a week or so earlier. One patient, exhausted by the ride home, encountered new pains and felt, for the first time, that he needed help getting into and out of bed.

"I was thrilled to get out of the hospital, but my euphoria didn't last long. The pain really started after I got home," he remembered.

Had this patient regressed? No, he was feeling the intensified pain that normally accompanies fatigue. Although he felt energetic when he got dressed that morning, the trip from the hospital wore him out. In the hospital, when he felt tired he got right into bed and rested. At home, the challenges and the distances were greater. Although his fatigue hit him as he got out of the car, he still had to walk to the house.

"The front path never seemed so long," he recalled.

Once inside, he went to lie down and suddenly found that task difficult, too.

"In the hospital, I had worked out this elaborate system of hanging on to the bed rail to ease myself into bed. I'd keep the bed tipped up and, once I was settled, I'd just push the electric button and adjust the angle to whatever position was comfortable. When I got home, I didn't have those contraptions, and I didn't realize how much I had depended on them. At home, my bed was too low and flat. Getting settled hadn't been so hard since the day after I left the ICU."

Another patient found it jolting to lose the insular quality of the hospital.

"In the hospital, I didn't have to worry about anything," she said. "Every morning, the nurse delivered my menu for the next day and I circled my choices. Then, like clockwork, the trays came and they were picked up. Not at home. My sister brought me home from the hospital and after she helped me get settled, she asked me what we should have for lunch. Lunch? Do I know? I had to think, 'What's in the house? Do I have tuna fish in the cupboard? Is there bread in the freezer? How can we have tuna fish without lettuce and tomatoes?' At that moment, it would have been no more difficult to negotiate an arms treaty with the Russians."

At home the walk from bed to bathroom is likely to be longer than in the hospital. At home, you are expected to shower, shave, and get dressed. While you will probably get up in the morning feeling full of energy, by the time you have accomplished a routine you normally don't give a second thought, half the morning will be gone and you will feel ready for a nap.

"I think the problems seemed worse at home because they were inconsistent with the feelings I associated with home. Resting every other minute in the hospital was normal enough. At home, I'm not accustomed to resting, and having to rest seemed to exaggerate my vulnerability," said a third patient.

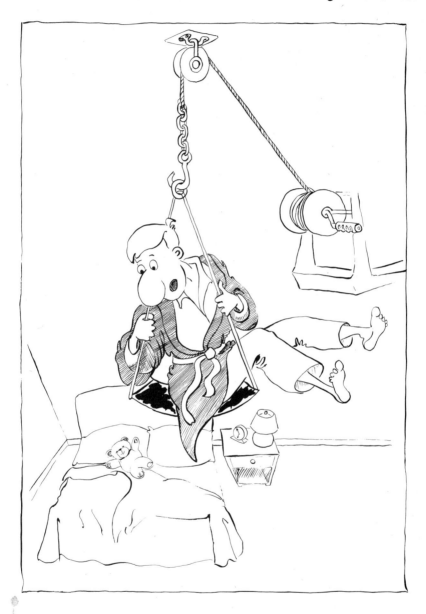

"At home, my bed was too low and flat."

"The weakness got to me," still another patient remembered. "For weeks, getting washed in the morning took forever. I had no ambition to do anything, and in the kitchen, I was helpless. I didn't have the strength to slice a carrot or open a can. A month after I was home, I got in the car for the first time to do an errand, and I didn't have enough strength in my arms to turn the wheel. I had to leave the car at the end of the driveway and go inside to call a friend to come and move it. Two weeks later, I was back at work, but I was still tired and needed to rest."

## Lingering Discomforts

You can expect a variety of unpleasant feelings after you are discharged. Pain in the incisions, rubbing of the sternum, and numbness in the chest may continue for weeks. Many patients complain of discomfort in their chests for months, especially when the barometer drops. In addition, sleeplessness, lack of appetite, and abdominal distress commonly persist, as do periodic feelings of anxiety, depression, and dependency. Some patients feel dizzy, frequently as a side effect of medication.

## Fatigue

For many, the most difficult aspect of recovery is the unique brand of fatigue characteristic of recuperation from surgery. Patients describe it as a bone-deep weariness that strikes without warning. Although most people perceive a marked increase in stamina after just a week at home, many of these same men and women contend that residual fatigue lingers for at least a year.

"One second I was fine, the next I was too tired," one patient recalled. "And when that exhaustion hit, I was no good for anything. Everything hurt more. My muscles quivered, and my nerves felt raw. It was terrible. I was told to rest before I felt tired, in other words to prevent fatigue. But when you're feeling fine and the fatigue comes without warning, that's hard to do."

That is hard to do, especially if you are impatient about recovering and eager to test your growing strength. Consequently, patients who feel fine typically drain their energy and then succumb to fatigue. For weeks life seems like a see-saw—one moment feeling fine, the next feeling wretched. In spite of steadily increasing levels of energy, every time fatigue and its companion pain hit, they are discouraging. "Will I ever recover?" patients understandably worry. Anticipating fatigue and resting before it strikes will reduce this see-sawing and the emotional havoc which accompanies it. If you can rest before you deplete your reservoir of energy, you will avoid untold frustration and demoralization.

## Depression and Irritability

Short-lived bouts of depression and irritability are virtually inevitable nevertheless, just as they were in the hospital. Emotional short fuses often accompany physical debilitation. In the first weeks at home, some patients become uncharacteristically dependent and childlike. Some are unable to make decisions as small as which movie to watch on the VCR. Many become unusually tense and sensitive. Intolerant of their own shortcomings and those of others, they can be unpleasant and difficult to live with. Little annoyances they normally ignore suddenly exasperate them: "Why are the television commercials so stupid? Damn it, the chicken is overcooked! I wish that neighbor would walk her dog somewhere else."

One patient, who said she had been accustomed to controlling her emotions since she had been a small girl, became angry and tearful after her surgery and stayed that way for months.

"I cried in church and I cried at the supermarket. I cried when I cooked, and I cried when I got into bed at night. I still don't really understand why I got so depressed," she said. "And angry! When my husband came home late, I got angry. When he came home early, I got angry, too. When he was sweet, I yelled at him for patronizing me, and when he wasn't, I cried because I thought he didn't care."

When faced with these feelings, patients sometimes withdraw. Some prefer not to socialize, as if they need to draw a protective shield around themselves so they can regain their strength and self-confidence. During this time they commonly cry with little provocation, although some stoics turn their depression inward because they cannot permit their feelings to show.

"Be patient when your dad gets withdrawn or surly," one former patient advised a young man whose father was about to undergo bypass surgery. "He will have to slow down every facet of his life. It's a difficult adjustment, and he won't be himself for a long time."

Ironically, this advice is particularly valid when it pertains to patients who felt little preoperative fear. Somehow, when patients are afraid beforehand, they have an easier time accepting the lengthy debilitation afterwards. Unconsciously they deduce that any procedure which could provoke so much apprehension must be serious enough to require a long and slow recuperation. Patients are also especially vulnerable to bouts of depression and irritability if they feel apprehensive about their well-being.

"I was relentlessly angry at my wife," recalled a patient whose short temper sent him back to the psychotherapist who had discharged him two years earlier. "I didn't realize I was really angry at my frailty and bad luck. Why me? What did I ever do to deserve a bad heart?"

Other patients are worried about dying. One asserted, "You're concerned about going through this again in a certain amount of time. You're concerned that even though everything feels fine, something is going to go wrong."

Another patient agreed, "I'm obsessed with the fear of dying." Though his surgery had taken place three months before he made this comment and although he was working full time, he acknowledged that questions about his mortality plagued him constantly.

A third patient put the same concerns slightly differently: "On some level, everyone knows they won't live forever. Since my surgery, though, questions about how well and how long I will live haunt me every day. I can force them to the back of my mind, but I can't make them go away."

While many patients learn to identify the causes of residual aches, some complain that they are forever uncertain. Persistent anxiety sends some back to their physicians repeatedly, and when an electrocardiogram confirms that all is well, they worry someone has made a mistake.

Understandably, when patients feel they are not recovering properly, they become more vulnerable to depression. And unfortunately, a variety of problems can linger or recur.

Memory loss and difficulty concentrating plague many bypass patients, sometimes for more than six months after they are home. Patients complain they cannot remember what they read, they forget people's names, they get confused easily, they lose their train of thought. Some reveal that, while they are talking, their minds suddenly go blank. Others say their mental processes have simply slowed down. These problems may be caused by medication, stress, hardening of the arteries, or a combination of factors.

It's a natural tendency for many people—especially when they feel vulnerable to illness—to presume the worst. "Memory difficulties? I must have had a stroke. Or maybe it's Alzheimer's disease. After all," patients could legitimately reason, "heart surgery can trigger a stroke, and I am at the age when lots of people show the first signs of Alzheimer's disease." Despite the tendency to draw conclusions like this, difficulties with thinking, concentrating, and remembering after heart surgery are almost always transient. Most patients who battle these difficulties report that they begin to subside after about six months, and within a year they are all but gone. These problems reflect permanent neurological damage in less than 1% of cases. Nevertheless, for people who have never had such difficulties before, they are understandably demoralizing.

While the problems persist, you can compensate by keeping notes and lists. A magnetic pad on the refrigerator, a tiny notebook for purse or pocket, pencils and paper in every room of the house are valuable crutches for two reasons. Most obviously, when ideas (even reminders to call Cousin Nancy or pick up a new drill bit at the hardware store) are committed to paper, they don't get forgotten. In addition, writing notes promotes learning. Just as school children often practice their spelling words by writing them over and over, when you write reminders to yourself, you may help to retrain your memory.

## Medical Complications

Occasionally, complications do arise or some degree of permanent disability lingers. A fifty-five-year-old veteran of two bypass operations was justifiably disheartened when shortness of breath prevented him from walking any appreciable distance. Another patient, who had recovered steadily for a month, was suddenly beset with postcardiotomy syndrome, characterized by fever, depression, aching, and chest pain frighteningly reminiscent of angina. Pleurisy and blood clots can impede recovery, and

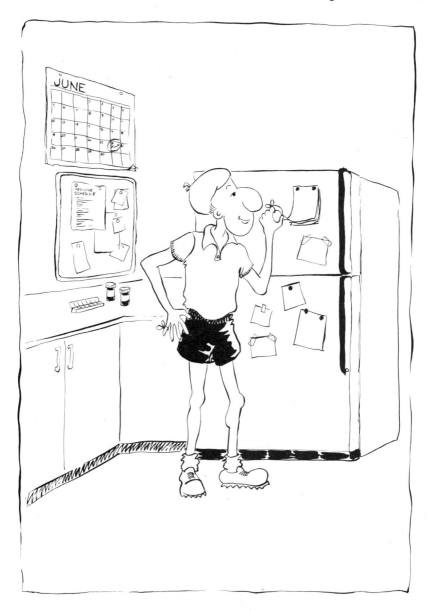

You can compensate by keeping notes and lists.

occasionally complications put patients back in the hospital.

Evelyn Samson was recovering slowly but steadily enough that she was able to maintain a positive outlook. Then she developed blood clots in her lung, which required her to be rehospitalized.

"You can't imagine how bleak the future looked at that point. Recovery had been hard, but I was staying with it, and then, I was back in the hospital. Oh, good Jesus, I was sure I would never get better," she lamented.

Though Evelyn Samson's clots were dissolved and she was released within a week, the setback was too much for her to cope with and she found herself unable to shake depression. Her cardiologist recommended short-term psychotherapy, which was effective, and Evelyn Samson was fully recovered, physically as well as emotionally, eight months later.

## Signs of Serious Depression

Our Miami Heart Institute Study found that patients recover emotionally at different rates just as they recover physically at different rates. Normal reactive depression may peak as late as three months after surgery. Almost always, it is a reflection of weakness and debilitation. It wanes decidedly as patients' vigor returns and they begin to assume more control over their lives. Some patients, however, continue to be plagued by depression in spite of solid physical recovery. Even months after surgery a few patients have trouble getting on with life. Some enjoy being invalids. They relish being nursed and pampered. Some who suffered from angina for years become so bound by fear that they are helpless. Some patients feel too listless to make love, plan an activity, or face the challenges of the day. They may feel estranged from their families, friends, colleagues, even from their former selves. They may see restaurant menus and television food commercials as ugly reminders of what they should not eat. They may interpret solicitous behavior by friends and colleagues as a measure of their compromised worth. They may become enraged because they feel their family and friends are patronizing them. These patients, together with those who fail to feel good despite their cardiologists' claims that they should, may be suffering long-term debilitating depression.

Profound depression demands attention by a trained mental health professional and, with professional help, can often be alleviated quickly. In the rare instance when patients are depressed because of permanent cardiac disability, psychotherapy can likewise be beneficial. While it cannot change the cardiac health picture, psychotherapy may enable patients to eat better, sleep more soundly, and feel more optimistic about their lives.

## Signs of Progress

Eager to put their surgery behind them, many patients assess recovery through tangible signs, literally measuring their progress in footsteps. As they walk farther and faster, they know they're getting better. Some identify progress with the easing of pain. *New York Times* journalist Douglass Cater reported that by the end of three weeks virtually all his pain was gone, leaving only residual aches in his rib cage, noticeable primarily at night and early in the morning. Other patients recall that the muscle pain in the shoulder blades subsided, or that the numbness in the chest diminished.

## Coping Strategies

In addition to tracking their progress, many patients make a conscious effort to cope. A number of patients find sustenance in God. Some who had always been religious rely heavily on faith. And some who had once rejected religion find themselves drawn to church or synagogue for the first time in many years.

Some patients meditate while others seek solitude on the beach or in the park. Still others rely on internal dialogue. One patient confided, "When I feel down, I make my intellectual self talk to my emotional self and say, 'You feel bad now, but you won't always feel this way.' Later, or the next day, when I am feeling better, my intellectual self reminds my emotional self, 'See, now you feel better. You might feel bad again, but it won't last.'"

Many patients attribute their recovery to the understanding and support they received from their families and friends. In a marriage where communication is good and mutual understanding solid, a husband and wife can relieve each other's stresses and grow closer in the process. Not every patient is married and not every marriage is good, however. One single man called upon his only cousin to support him through surgery, and found that their relationship deepened because his cousin felt needed. Another single patient set up a schedule for her friends.

"I was conscious of not overburdening anyone, and I figured that my friends would appreciate specific requests. So I gave everyone an assignment. I always had company when I wanted it, and there was always someone to go to the grocery store or cook dinner."

Some patients found comfort comparing notes with other patients and, after they recovered, found ongoing strength in peer support groups. After their recovery, several began serving as peer advisors to help other patients through their surgery and recovery.

"It helps to know that other people are feeling what you are feeling," one advocate of peer support groups asserted.

While support from others is invaluable, the bulk of the responsibility for recovery lies with you. Inherent in this responsibility is a positive attitude and a commitment to work hard. As Barbara Friedman, clinical nurse specialist, tells her discharge classes, "You may have ten minutes every day for a pity party. No more. It's self-defeating."

One patient, with a history of cancer, osteoporosis, and more than a dozen major operations, claimed that a positive attitude enabled her to recover from heart surgery despite serious complications.

"I push, that's all," she summarized. "I get up and I walk even though I know that I'll be in agony when I get home. When I couldn't walk because of leg problems, I rode a stationary bike. Sometimes, I get blue and I cry. 'I don't believe it,' I tell my husband. 'Here's another problem. I'd like to wake up just once and feel fine.' So he sits beside me and strokes my back and tells me, 'You're entitled.' But before you know it he'll remind me of someone who has worse trouble. Then I think, 'Well, I survived this,' and I feel better."

Several years after her surgery, she still had many medical problems, but she did not dwell on them. "No day is boring. Our travel and activity are limited because of my health," she admitted, "but we always find adventure. We walk in different places, we drive to different destinations, we explore new stores and museums."

Setting a purpose or a goal helped many patients keep a positive attitude during the difficult weeks. One patient planned the retirement he had looked forward to for years. He started painting, made travel plans, and set up a part-time consulting business. Other retired people prepared to invest their energies in a hobby, volunteer work, activities with friends, or organizations. After six weeks or so, when they were able to do the activities they planned, they discovered the diversion took their minds off their bodies and put a better sense of balance back into their lives. For patients who had not yet retired, returning to work was often a panacea. It kept them busy, distracted them from their discomforts, and reaffirmed their sense of worth.

As one patient, who returned to work six weeks after surgery, put it, "I don't have time to think about my aches and pains."

In the early weeks of recovery, patients are commonly egocentric and excessively alert to every ache and twinge, but this preoccupation ultimately fades. As the weeks stretch into months and patients feel stronger, most let go of their fixation with their health and mortality. One patient, who had a coronary one September and bypass surgery the following January, returned to his job as a mechanic in July, rejoined his bowling team in August, and bowled his first 200 game of the season in September. Six years later, he was vigorous and active. Although he and his wife remained dedicated members of their hospital's support group, they spent little time ruminating about his well-being.

In these later months, many patients discover that life is better than it ever has been. Many boast their surgery made them appreciate life in a refreshing new way. Some become less driven, more capable of relaxing and enjoying leisure time. Some proclaim they have become motivated less by guilt and obligation, more by desire and genuine interest. Some claim they have learned to live with greater joy; they are more candid and forthright, and they appreciate their loved ones more.

Within a year after surgery—and it may take that long—most patients feel they have changed for the better in some way. Many, many patients feel reborn and rejuvenated. Experiencing more than a change in philosophy, these people discover reservoirs of energy that make them feel ten, twenty years younger. They are jubilant to be rid of their angina, to be able to eat, walk, swim, and run without pain. Many claim that, with a new appreciation for their loved ones, their marriages and family lives have improved. Many feel their experience has given them more insight into themselves. Some have acquired greater religious faith.

One patient, celebrating the first anniversary of his bypass, exclaimed how grateful he felt to have had the surgery. "To think that I'm alive! How lucky I am. I'm fortunate that medical science is as sophisticated as it is. I was lucky to have my surgeon and to have recovered. And now, I'm thrilled because I feel so good."

## Points to Remember

❑ Gradually you will grow stronger and more self-confident.

❑ Continue the work of recovery diligently.

❑ Anticipate fatigue and rest before it strikes.

❑ Call your designated medical liaison when you have questions or concerns.

❑ Utilize relaxation techniques, meditation, self-dialogue, and other coping techniques.

❑ Compensate for memory loss by making lists.

❑ Give your family and friends specific requests for help and support.

Chapter Seven

# PRESCRIPTION FOR RECOVERY

Recovering from heart surgery requires patience and perseverance. It is aided by breaking down overwhelming problems into smaller, more manageable components; putting depression into perspective; and remembering that, while one day might look bleak, the next is bound to be brighter. This chapter is a manual for this process, with detailed attention to the first weeks. In all instances where these guidelines differ from your physician's instructions, defer to your physician. If you have questions about any of these instructions, talk with your doctor.

## Arranging for Help

During at least your first week home, you should have someone with you most of the time, for many of your tasks will require help. If your spouse works, this first week at home—not the week you were in the hospital—is the best time for him or her to take off. Sometimes spouses, particularly husbands, feel threatened by this kind of responsibility. If so, call on someone else. If you live alone, you'll need someone to stay with you as well. A friend, a grown son or daughter, even a hired practical nurse will do, but you should not be alone for more than a couple of hours at a time. If your only choice is a married child with a family of his or her own who lives in a distant city, consider imposing. Having your son or daughter with you will solve your practical problems. In addition, it might give you the opportunity for a uniquely meaningful visit. In the atmosphere of recovery, where you need help and your child can meet your needs, new, long-lasting bonds often form. At the end of the week, when you kiss each other good-bye, you are likely to discover your relationship has strengthened, your closeness deepened.

## Clothing

For the trip home and for the next couple of weeks, choose clothing that is easy to put on and comfortable to wear. Women often find that wearing a bra, even for sleeping, helps keep their breasts from pulling against their incisions. Some women prefer front-closing bras because they are easier to fasten, while others choose bras that close in the back because they are less irritating to the healing scar. Men sometimes complain that button-down shirts irritate their scars as does the hair growing in on their chests. Patients who have been particularly bothered by their healing incisions have devised a variety of ingenious contraptions to protect them. Some have tried dry gauze bandages, though they readily admit that putting tape onto the itchy stubble of new chest hair is less than satisfactory. Some have experimented with thin, self-adhering sanitary napkins which they stick to their clothing. Try using one pad over the scar as a bandage. Alternatively, affix one pad on either side of the scar to form a protective channel. Sometimes women, as well as men, find comfort in a plain cotton T-shirt worn as an undershirt. Most patients simply opt for pullover shirts in a soft fabric.

Beyond comfort, appearance matters, not for visitors but for you. Looking good will help lift your mood while it subtly reminds you that, although you are newly home from the hospital, you are not sick; you are recovering from surgery. Choose attractive clothing in appealing colors. Men, shave every day and splash on your favorite after-shave cologne. Women, if you enjoy wearing makeup, put it on every day. If you get your hair washed and set, arrange for someone to do that for you soon after you come home. If you blow your hair dry, arrange for someone to help you with that as often as you normally wash your hair. Allotting extra time and making special arrangements are well worth their trouble. If you ask friends and relatives to help you with these and other specific tasks, they will probably be grateful; knowing how they can help you will make them feel wanted and needed.

## Support Stockings

Continue to wear your support stockings for two to three weeks at home. You may take these off to sleep at night and to bathe, but they should be put on before you get out of bed in the morning. You'll need help with this task. It's a struggle, and your incision has not healed enough for you to manage it alone.

To support your legs properly, your elastic stockings must lie smoothly. Wrinkles act as rubber bands and will cut off your circulation. To help your elastic stockings do their job, keep your legs elevated whenever you are sitting, and remember not to cross your legs.

## Activity Schedule

For at least five to six weeks following your discharge, recuperation will be a full-time job. By balancing activity and rest, you can fill the entire day. Like any job, recuperation has its challenges and its drudgery. It includes work that is best done alone and work that benefits from team cooperation. Remember that, although five weeks can feel like an eternity, especially when those weeks are marked by discomforts and depression, this period will end. Your strength will return. You will feel better. In the meantime, respect disability.

If you go to bed and try to sleep more than once during the day, you will probably have greater difficulty sleeping at night. Try to get as many of hours sleep at night as you normally do. If you find you must stay up late one night, try to nap earlier in the day. Force yourself to exercise despite lethargy. Getting up and getting going will help raise your spirits and spark some energy.

**Day of Discharge:** When you get home from the hospital, you will probably be so tired you will want to lie down. Even if you don't feel tired, rest for an hour when you first get home. Then resume whatever schedule you were following your last day or so in the hospital.

**Duration of the First Week at Home:** Take pain medications according to your discharge instructions. Applying moist heat will also relieve pain. If you can, use an electric fomentation unit (brand name Thermophore), a heating pad designed to create moist heat by utilizing the moisture in your body. If you don't have one and can't obtain one, use a damp towel beneath a heating pad shielded with a heat-resistant plastic cover. You'll need help wetting the towel and wringing it out. If you attempt this task yourself, you will strain your chest incision, so ask someone else to do it for you.

If you are taking medicine for pain, plan to begin exercising forty-five minutes to an hour after your pill. Continue your physical therapy exercises once a day. Do your breathing exercises four times a day. Walk in the house four times a day. It's important to cool down after exercise so your heart rate slows gradually. To cool down, breathe slowly and deeply. While sitting down, point your toes then flex your feet ten times. Bend your knees and straighten your legs ten times. Rest before showering.

Since exercising and eating tax the heart, you should rest for one hour after meals and half an hour between activities, preferably *not* in bed. A recliner is ideal. If you don't have one and can't borrow one, try a comfortable lounge chair or couch. Remember, however, that the lower and flatter you put yourself, the harder it will be to get up and down independently.

The bone incision in your chest, like a broken bone, takes five weeks to heal. During this time, *do not* lift or push anything that weighs more than ten to fifteen pounds. *Do not* vacuum, mow the lawn, move furniture, lift a baby, carry groceries or suitcases, or reach for objects on a shelf above your head. In addition, *do not* try to unscrew a stubborn jar, open a sticking window, or perform any other task which requires a similar struggle.

Activities like these will keep your chest incision from healing. To make yourself more self-sufficient in the kitchen, have someone move dishes and glasses so that they are no higher than shoulder level. In addition, unstack pots and pans so you don't have to lift a heavy pile in order to get to the one on the bottom.

When you first get home, everything you do will take longer than usual. Showering, dressing, eating, exercising, and resting will consume nearly the entire day. By the end of the first week at home, a typical day might look like this:

8:00   Wake up, wash and have breakfast.
8:30   Rest with a morning T.V. show; do breathing exercises.
9:30   Shower, get help putting on elastic stockings.
9:45   Rest with the morning newspaper.
10:15  Shave or put on your makeup; get dressed.
10:45  Rest with Duke Ellington; do breathing exercises.
11:15  Physical therapy.
12:00  Lunch.
12:30  Rest with the afternoon news; perhaps you'll doze.
2:30   Walk; cool down.
3:30   Rest with Agatha Christie; do breathing exercises.
4:00   Entertain guests for one hour.

| | |
|---|---|
| 5:00 | Rest with the *National Geographic*. |
| 5:30 | Prepare a martini and make the salad for dinner. |
| 6:00 | Dinner. |
| 6:30 | Rest with the evening news; do breathing exercises. |
| 7:30 | Play a round of poker with some friends. |
| 9:30 | Bed; remove elastic stockings. |

Some patients complain that recovery is unbearably monotonous. If you use your resting time creatively, it is likely to seem less dreary. Take advantage of this time to think through home repair projects you've been planning for years, dictate letters to your secretary, study new cookbooks and learn the principles of good nutrition, get on the phone and make contact with a friend whom you haven't spoken to in months. As time goes on, the length of your activities will increase, and you will need to rest fewer times each day.

**Second Week:** Continue resting one hour after each meal, half an hour after each activity. Continue breathing exercises four times a day and physical therapy once a day.

You may take walks outside now when the weather is mild. Be careful to keep your incision covered; sunlight will damage this tender new skin. Begin with no more than one block once a day. Remember, however far you walk away from home, you must return the same distance, and fatigue often strikes without warning. Test your stamina and increase your distance gradually. By the end of this week, you should be doing four blocks (two blocks each way) or one-fourth of a mile. Choose flat terrain. In the summer, walk in the evening or early in the morning to avoid intense heat and sun. In the winter, choose the middle of the day to avoid extreme cold or wind. Since hills, wind, heat, cold, and sun make the heart work harder, you may have to continue walking indoors for a second week. Alternatively, you can spend your exercise time riding a stationary bicycle at low tension. Try reading a book, watching television, or listening to music while you ride to help pass the time. Under no circumstances is inclement weather an excuse not to exercise. Continue cool-down exercises, and rest before showering. If exercise produces pain, stop, rest, and consult your doctor.

Always take and record your pulse before walking and exercising, then again immediately upon finishing. Pressing lightly but firmly with your index and middle fingers, find the radial artery on the palm side of your wrist. Never use your thumb to take your pulse since the thumb also has a pulse which can confuse your count. Count the number of beats for six seconds, then add a zero to your number to determine your heart rate for one minute. If you have trouble finding your pulse, you can purchase a mechanical pulse meter, sold at sporting goods stores. These vary in design, capability, accuracy, and price, beginning at about $70.00.

Your heart rate during exercise should be at least ten beats per minute higher than your resting heart rate but no higher than 120. Use your pulse rate as a guide for increasing your workout; if your heart rate rises more than thirty beats per minute, do not increase the duration and vigor of your regime. As your stamina increases, your present routine will raise your heart rate less. When your exercising heart rate rises less than thirty beats per minute, you can safely increase your challenges.

Your pulse should return to its resting rate within fifteen minutes of finishing your workout. If it exceeds 120 during exercise or fails to slow sufficiently within fifteen minutes, consult your doctor.

This week and always, try to set a consistent time each day for exercising. Doing so will help put structure in your day and assure that the day doesn't slip by without this all-important activity. Use good judgment to strike a healthy balance between increasing your activity level and avoiding fatigue.

This week you may begin to climb stairs. Take them slowly, one step at a time, and remember to breathe deeply. Resist the inclination to hold your breath. (See section on physical therapy exercises below.)

You may take short rides as a passenger in the car, get your hair cut, visit your favorite hardware store. (Be sure to wear your seat belt even if you are going only to the corner drug store; a minor accident could ram you into the dashboard and injure your healing breastbone.)

During inclement weather, consider riding to a local mall for your walks. Increasingly, malls are opening their corridors half an hour or so before the stores open so walkers can get their exercise. Don't forget to cool down. Try walking with a friend, then stopping for a cup of tea or a glass of juice to rest up before the car ride home.

**Third Week:** Continue to rest for one hour after meals and for thirty minutes between activities. Continue physical therapy, breathing exercises, and walking. Don't forget to cool down and rest before showering. By the end of this week, you should be up to eight to twelve blocks. During this week, you may go out to dinner with friends, take in a movie, plan other short adventures.

If your legs are not swollen, you may stop wearing your elastic stockings.

You may also resume sexual intercourse. (See section on sex below.)

This week you should begin to massage your chest incision with lotion. (See section on bathing and caring for your incision below.)

**Fourth Week:** Continue to rest for one hour after meals and half an hour between activities. You may stop your breathing exercises after this week, but continue your physical therapy and increase your walking up to sixteen to twenty blocks, or one mile. With the exception of strenuous exertion, resume all normal activities.

With your physician's approval, you may be able to start driving this week. Since you may still be weaker than you think and your reflexes may still be slower than normal, test your mettle cautiously. At first, take short trips on quiet streets free from heavy traffic. For the first several times you drive, have someone in the passenger's seat who can take the wheel if you feel tired.

If a hospital in your area offers a cardiac rehabilitation program, this might be the week for you to begin. For the first couple of months, you should attend three times a week.

**Fifth Week:** Continue to rest for one hour after meals and half an hour between activities. Continue your physical therapy and increase the distance you are walking until you reach forty blocks, or two miles. Dedicate yourself to walking two miles or doing a comparable aerobic exercise every day for the rest of your life. If you find exercise boring, plan to do it with a friend. Call your peer support group (see section on peer support groups below) and get a buddy. Plan different walks each day. Explore the new housing development, a different shopping mall, the local parks.

With your physician's permission, you may return to work for about four hours a day. In two more weeks, you will be able to return full time if your physician permits.

Continue to increase your activities gradually. Continue to anticipate fatigue, and rest before it strikes. Even in the coming months, avoid booking social engagements on heavy business days. Avoid heavy meals. Strive for moderation. Remember, recovery may take a full year.

## Physical Therapy Exercises

Physical therapy exercises prevent circulatory disorders, increase mobility, and help improve stamina. In many hospitals, physical therapists work individually

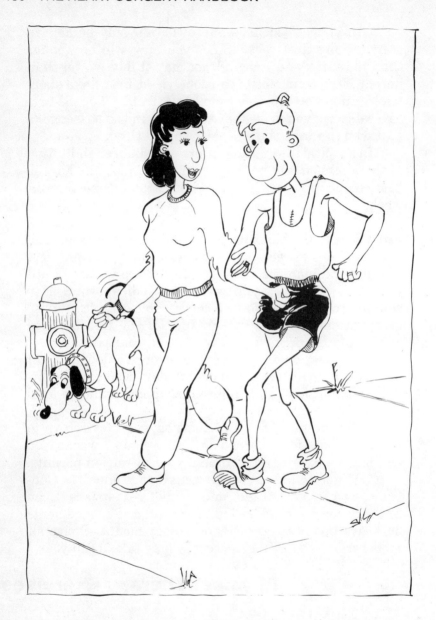

If you find excercise boring, plan to do it with a friend.

with patients on a daily basis, gradually increasing the patients' physical challenges. Before patients are discharged, their physical therapists give them a regimen of exercises, together with suggestions and admonitions, to follow at home.

If you received a physical therapy regime, follow it. Otherwise you might try this one, building your tolerance gradually. Do these exercises once a day at least one hour after eating or half an hour after a preceding activity. If chest pain occurs during exercise, stop and rest for fifteen minutes. If the chest pain continues, call your doctor. When you exercise, be careful not to hold your breath or you will prevent the exchange of carbon dioxide for oxygen when you need it most. Counting out loud will keep you breathing in spite of the instinctive tendency not to.

1. *Lying face up on a bed (the floor is too hard), slide one leg out to the side, and slide it back. Do the same with the other leg. Repeat the pattern four more times.*

2. *Lying face up on the bed with your arms at your side, raise one arm and reach over your head. Bring your arm back to your side. Then do the same with the other arm. Repeat this pattern four more times.*

3. *Lying in the same position, raise one knee as close to your chest as possible. At the same time, reach for your knees with both hands. Return to the starting position and do the same exercise lifting the other knee. Repeat this sequence four more times.*

4. *Sitting on the edge of the bed and supporting yourself with both hands behind you, straighten one leg, then return to the original*

*position. Then do the same with the other leg. Repeat the pattern four more times.*

5. *Sitting on the edge of the bed, make a fist and bend both arms toward your chest as though you were going to beat your chest. Working one arm at a time, straighten your elbow and extend your arm out to the side. Return it to the original position. Repeat the sequence five times with each arm.*

6. *Sitting on the edge of the bed, resume the original position of the preceding exercise. Twist from the waist up as far to the left as possible. Repeat the movement ten times. Then twist to the right ten times.*

7. *Standing on the floor and supporting yourself against the wall if necessary, rock onto your tiptoes and then back down. Begin with ten repetitions, and when that feels easy, increase by two repetitions every three to four days.*

8. *Standing up and supporting yourself comfortably, bend your knees gently; then return to a straight-leg position. Follow the repetition instructions in the last exercise.*

9. *Perform the trunk twist described above but in a standing position. Follow the repetition instructions in the preceding exercise.*

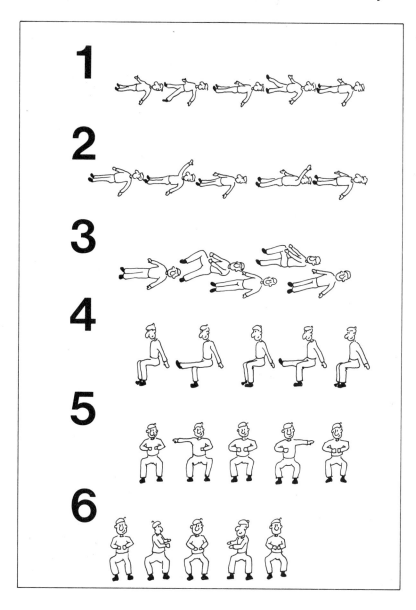

Add the following three exercises no sooner than ten weeks after being home, as late as twelve weeks if necessary:

10. *Sitting on the bed with your legs gently spread before you, reach for your right toes with your left hand. Then reach for your left toes with your right hand. Begin with ten repetitions on each side, and when you feel ready, increase this sequence by two counts every three to four days.*

11. *Sitting on the bed with your hands behind you on the bed for support, lift your right leg slightly, slowly swing it as far to the right as you can, and then bring it back. Do the same with the other leg. Increase the repetitions for each leg as in preceding exercise.*

12. *Standing on the floor with your feet slightly apart and your hands on your hips, extend your right arm over your head, and bend your trunk to the left as far as possible. Return to an upright position and repeat. Then switch, extending your left arm over your head and bending your trunk to the right as far as possible. Increase repetitions as in the preceding exercise.*

The following suggestions may also be helpful:

If you feel stiff when you wake up in the morning or after a nap, do some of your physical therapy exercises to limber up. Fight the postsurgical inclination to stoop by making a conscious effort to think about good posture. Try to hold your head up and your back straight. Tape a note on the bathroom mirror and refrigerator door to help you remember. If you find you're hunching up your shoulders, you're probably tensing muscles in your torso unnecessarily. Try to keep your shoulders loose without stooping

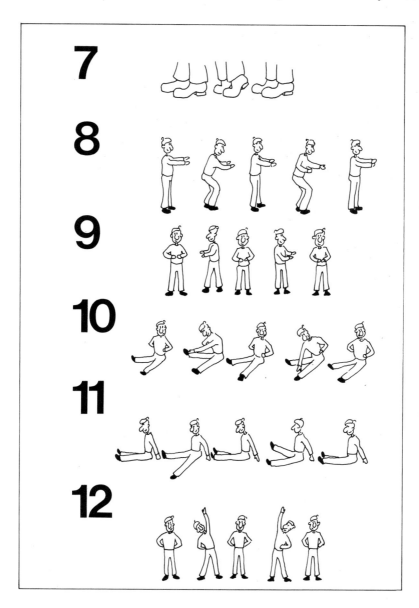

forward. If the surgery has confused your muscle memory and you can't tell whether you're standing straight, check your posture in the mirror.

Ask your physician when you can resume sports. Also, discuss whether, at some future date, you should aim for a higher target heart rate during aerobic exercise. Get a firm sense of how high your heart rate should go, how long it should stay there, and what your resting heart rate should be. Then you can work out an exercise regime that is emotionally satisfying as well as physically therapeutic.

## Drugs

It is important to know what drugs you take, what each drug does, what its potential side effects and dangers are, and what precautions to take to avert them. You should go over your medications and detailed instructions for taking them with your physician. Run through the drugs you took routinely or occasionally before surgery: antihistamines, antacids, and other over-the-counter preparations as well as any prescription drugs. Ask about using alcohol, driving, and operating machinery in relation to your new drugs. In addition, find out whether sexual impotence or depression ever occurs as a side effect.

Remember that each person metabolizes and reacts to drugs individually. Balancing drugs effectively is often a matter of trial and error, and it may take some juggling before your physician finds the best combination of drugs in the ideal dosages for you. Since adjustments may need to be made, pay attention to your reactions and don't be shy about calling your physician if you are concerned about your medications.

Keep a chart of your medications posted in the kitchen or bathroom and diligently note when you take each one. This will help you keep track until your medication schedule becomes routine. If you miss a dose, do not double up the next time. Do not stop taking any medication because you think it's causing a problem. If you have any questions or concerns, consult your doctor.

## Bathing and Caring for Your Incision

You may begin to shower twenty-four hours after your staples or stitches come out. Showering, you may discover, is tiring. Avoid steamy hot showers as they will strain your heart and drain your energy. At least at first, it's a good idea to have a stool in the shower so you can sit. Have your spouse or someone else nearby so you can call for help if you feel tired. Keep soap off your incision for the first three days. Sit on the toilet seat cover or a hamper to dry yourself. Pat your incision dry. Plan to rest before shaving, putting on your makeup, or getting dressed.

Caring for your incision will help to relieve itching and minimize the width of your scar. If butterfly bandages were placed across your incision, you may remove them in three days. Beginning the third week you are home, massage your chest in the following manner:

Coat your hands with skin lotion or baby oil. Place one hand on either side of your incision and gently massage the skin beside the incision in circles toward the incision. Repeat this practice five times a day.

Two weeks later, add circles away from your incision. Now you are massaging both toward the incision and away from it at least four times a day.

Another two weeks later, begin massaging directly over the incision. Keep up these massages four to five times a day for at least three months.

Pay attention to your incision as you massage it or shower. If you notice any new fluid draining from your incision or if your incision appears newly red or swollen, call your doctor. You should also be alert for other signs of infection, namely fever, increased sensitivity, or heat at the site of the incision. Remember that some discomfort emanating from the incision is normal and may continue for more than a year.

## Cardiac Rehabilitation

Attending a cardiac rehabilitation laboratory is an excellent alternative to walking. In the lab, patients wear cardiac monitors and perform their exercise routines under the guidance of physical therapists. The monitors will reassure you that the exercise is not harmful, and chatting informally with the staff will help to eliminate nagging fears. In addition, many patients value the peer support and social contact that accompany exercising with others. They find that company makes exercising more enjoyable and helps them establish new habits they will practice for life. The cardiac rehab lab is also a good place to compare notes and discover that your experiences resemble other patients'.

## Insomnia

Patients commonly complain that they have difficulty sleeping for several weeks after surgery. If you have trouble, eliminate caffeine from your diet. Eliminate alcohol as well; although alcohol has the tendency to induce sleepiness initially, its long-term effects disrupt sleep. Avoid napping during the day; make an effort to go to bed at the same time every night and get up early in the morning.

Many patients find establishing a bedtime ritual helps to turn off the mind and prepare it for sleep. One patient began his sequence at 11:00 every night. He took a warm bath, drank a cup of sleepy-time tea, got into bed, read his favorite psalm, turned on a relaxation tape, and before too many nights had passed, discovered he was asleep before the tape finished. Although the warm bath, hot tea, prayer, and soothing tape may have helped to relax him, the consistency of the ritual was probably the most important ingredient. If you like classical music, incorporate it into your ritual. If you like hot milk, that's fine, too. But so are apples and club soda, so long as you have them every night.

If insomnia persists, discuss it with your physician. Your problem may be medical, and your physician may want to treat it with medication. But before you resort to sleeping pills unnecessarily, try the suggestions above. They can't hurt, and they just might solve the problem.

# Diet

In the early days and weeks after surgery, don't be surprised if your taste for food is gone. Anesthesia and medications can make food taste unduly salty, unduly sweet, downright unpalatable. Until your appetite comes back, eat whatever you please so long as you maintain a well-balanced, nutritious diet.

Once your appetite comes back, however, it's time to reduce salt and lower fats. This is the moment so many patients dread. "How will I survive without chocolate cake?" many wonder. Others worry that, since they are on a restricted diet, no one will invite them to dinner parties anymore. It's true that for many patients a low-fat, low-cholesterol diet represents a dramatic change. And often that change feels like a punishment, a life-long sentence of tasteless, boring food. The prohibitions all but scream at you: no fatty meats, no cream cheese, no sausage, no potato chips.

Instead of dwelling on what you cannot have, approach

your new eating plan as an adventure, and the entire picture will change. If you're a fried chicken and potatoes fan, roll skin-free chicken pieces in potato buds, drizzle them with cholesterol-free oil, and bake them. If you seek exotic fare, enjoy the temptations of Pasta Raphael, a sauce made from tomatoes, fresh basil, and artichoke hearts; grilled swordfish steaks marinated in lime juice and saki seasoned with soy sauce, fresh garlic, fresh ginger, and cayenne pepper; fresh poached peaches with fresh raspberry sauce. These low-fat recipes come from popular cookbooks *(Silver Palate, Frog Commissary,* and *Mastering the Art of French Cooking)* and illustrate that healthful dining can be wonderful. To help you get adjusted, try these tips:

Think creativity. When chicken gets boring, prepare a turkey breast. Instead of seasoning with standard salt, pepper, and garlic, mix up a marinade made from a little oil, a splash of soy sauce, pepper, ginger, orange marmalade, and grated rind of an orange. Marinate the turkey breast overnight. Bake it—better yet, cook it in the microwave, then brown it under the broiler. You'll have a succulent turkey breast with a subtle but penetrating orange flavor. If you like it, experiment with other marinades for chicken, turkey, and fish. Play with tomato juice mixed with Italian spices—thyme, oregano, and basil. Try wines, brandy, and soups as marinade bases. Get to know curry, cardamom, and cumin. Learn to stir-fry. Make a thick, meatless marinara sauce using finely chopped onion, garlic, green pepper, celery, and carrots; season with lots of Italian spice.

Think substitution. You can often lower the fat content of recipes without sacrificing flavor. You can saute in a fraction of the fat that most recipes specify, and you can choose safflower oil or olive oil instead of butter or oils higher in saturated fats. Use cholesterol-free oil and skim milk instead of butter and cream to make a white sauce; use corn starch mixed with water to thicken defatted drippings for gravy; use ground turkey or veal instead of ground beef; reduce salt and salty ingredients like soy sauce gradually, all the while compensating with a greater abundance of herbs and spices; replace caffeinated drinks with decaffeinated equivalents. Since caffeine stimulates the heart, drink no more than three cups of regular coffee, tea, or cola a day.

Think contribution. If you sense you're being overlooked on the dinner party circuit, suggest to a good friend a pot-luck supper where everyone brings a dish to share. If you bring a sufficient quantity of a delicious low-fat, low-cholesterol dish, everyone will help themselves from the same serving bowl and no one will look like an outcast. And while your discretion may guide you away from some of the choices, you will certainly be able to enjoy others.

Think research. The list of recommended foods has changed recently. Olive oil has joined the recommended list. So, happily, have shellfish—lobster, shrimp, scallops, and crabmeat. Researchers have discovered that these foods contain Omega-3 fatty acids that reduce cholesterol. Discover the Tufts University nutrition newsletter, where the latest findings are promptly reported. Spend some time in your local book store or library studying both specialty and general cookbooks. With more and more people—those who have heart disease and those who want to prevent it—converting to healthful lifestyles, there has been a surge of healthful recipes. Jane Brody and Craig Claiborne, to name just two authors, have devoted books to the subject. Other cookbook writers have included increasing numbers of low-fat recipes among their collections. Set yourself the goal of trying one new recipe each week, and before long you'll not only be eating more healthfully, but more adventurously as well.

Think adventure. Many cuisines, notably the Oriental ones, are inherently low in fat. Try a Thai or Japanese restaurant. Visit a pasta restaurant or a cafe specializing in nouvelle cuisine. Classic French restaurants, obviously, offer relatively few low-fat selections, but even there, you are bound to find a simple but delicious coq au vin or poached fish.

Think elegance. You're well and you deserve to celebrate. Take out the good silver and china. Enjoy some wine in a delicate stemmed glass. (Unless you are taking blood thinners, or your doctor says otherwise, you may have up to two ounces of hard liquor or three ounces of sweet wine or five ounces of dry wine or ten ounces of beer a day.)

One last word on diet: No one ever said you could never have another piece of chocolate cake. First of all, don't think in terms of never. Just think in terms of today. And yes, you may splurge occasionally. Occasionally. As time goes on and you discover new delicacies and treats, however, chances are you'll want to less and less.

## Sex

Yes, you can and should make love if you want to. It cannot damage your heart, disturb your bypasses, or hurt your incision. Are you afraid to have sex? Probably. Is your partner scared? Undoubtedly. Nearly everyone—patients and partners alike—worries about the ability to perform, about hurting the heart, about being too worried to enjoy the encounter, about how a bypass scar alters sex appeal. Sometimes patients don't even realize they are worried, but somehow, mysteriously, they might discover they have lost their desire and their potency. If you used to have angina, which cried stop every time you approached orgasm, you probably have been conditioned by fear. Can worries like these ruin your experience? Maybe. But there are things you can do to protect it. If you can, talk to your partner honestly and openly. Some people have trouble doing this. If you are one of them, communicate in whatever manner you communicate best, and remember that intercourse is only one facet of verbal and tactile communication that spells care, consideration, concern. Ideally, you and your partner have a tender, touching communication, which comforted you before surgery, in the ICU, and frequently since then. Even during your first week at home, there is no reason why kissing and caressing can't be a part of your time together watching television, listening to music, or talking in bed before you fall asleep. Sharing the worries which you and your partner are bound to have is part of this close communication. In bed, as in every other life arena, festering fear invites trouble. No one describes this as poignantly as Martha Weinman Lear in *Heartsounds*:

> It seemed crucial that he not know how scared I was. Lying there silently, as though my mind were on my pleasure. Watching him in the half-light that came from the bathroom, seeing the fingers pressed so slyly against his carotid artery, wondering what the pressure told him. Feeling his rhythm, the contact so sweet, and hearing him breathe heavily like that, and wondering if it was okay or too much. Then feeling his body go still. Was he all right? Did I dare ask?
>
> I felt poised at the edge of an irredeemable mistake. It would be dreadful to make him feel like an invalid here, of all places, impulse gone, confidence gone, good-bye, and maybe for good.
>
> And yet it might be even more dangerous to say nothing. For his body was in motion again now, and what if he was feeling pain, denying it, pushing himself to perform?
>
> "Do you want to rest a moment?" I whispered.
>
> Wrong. He made a sound like a sob and fell away from me, and we lay silent, not touching in any way.

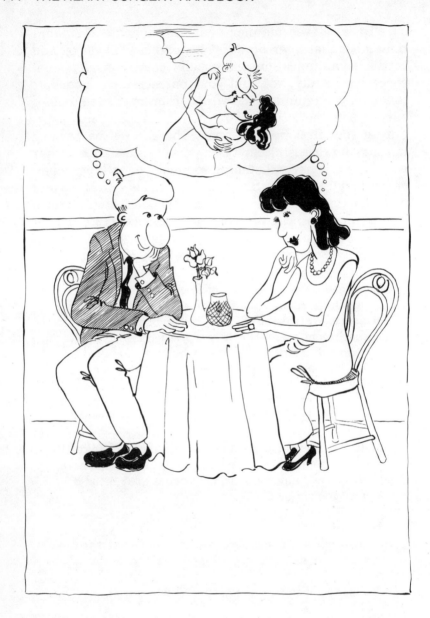

Don't rush. Be tender. Have fun.

Surely, candid communication can help avert a disaster like this one. So can testing yourself. If you can walk up two flights of stairs without panting, feeling exhausted, or experiencing pain, you won't have trouble during sex. If you still feel apprehensive, consider masturbation. Pay attention to the way your heart pounds, your breathing speeds up, and your body feels hot. These are normal feelings.

Choose the time and place for your sexual encounters carefully. Make sure you are well rested and that you have time to rest afterwards. Wait two to three hours after a heavy meal or alcoholic beverage. Adjust the thermostat in the room so the temperature is comfortable. Pick a moment when you and your partner are feeling good about yourselves and about each other; this is not the time to use sex to resolve an argument, dispel anxiety, or melt away hostility.

Don't rush. Be tender. Have fun. Light a candle. Play soft music. Engage in all your favorite foreplays and afterplays. If you like oral sex, by all means, indulge. If you enjoy caressing each other with baby oil, go right ahead. If you're nervous or worried, tell your partner and invite your partner to do likewise. Consider tempering anxiety with humor. Choose a comfortable position which does not strain your chest incision or hamper free breathing. Try lying on your side facing one another, or entering from behind. Men, try lying on your back with your partner on top; you will probably find the missionary position the most uncomfortable.

Despite good intentions, satisfactory sexual encounters may take some time. Surgery does lower the libido temporarily, as does anxiety. Be patient; be understanding. If impotence or lack of desire persists, discuss the problem with your doctor. Many cases of impotence are caused by medical problems that can be solved. Often these problems occur as side effects of medication, and altering your prescriptions may do the trick. Do not stop taking your medicine on your own, however. In addition, consult your physician if your heartbeat and breathing remain rapid for more than twenty minutes after orgasm, if you experience chest pain during intercourse, if you correlate insomnia with intercourse, or if you feel unusually tired the next day.

If difficulty with sex persists or if you find your doctor cannot help (some feel uncomfortable talking about sex), consider consulting a sex therapist. A few sessions may reveal the source of your difficulties and offer you specific suggestions for managing them.

One admonition: Having faced their mortality, many patients feel compelled to reevaluate their lives and, in this spirit, sometimes contemplate changing their sexual partners. If you are married or involved in a steady relationship, resist the urge. Affairs under these circumstances often promote guilt and anxiety, which put increased stress on the heart. The medical community makes the point with this stale joke:

Noticing a look of worry on his patient's face, the cardiologist asked, "What seems to be troubling you?"

The patient blushed and stammered, "Sex, doctor. Will I ever have sex again?"

"Of course," the cardiologist reassured him. "But only with your wife. We don't want you getting too excited."

## Peer Support Groups

Peer support groups have been developed in many hospitals where heart surgery is performed. Usually, the best programs are those designed and supported by the professionals who take care of heart surgery patients. These peer support organizations hold monthly meetings, during which patients at various stages of recovery convene to share experiences, listen to speakers on various pertinent subjects, and make new friends. Some patients find these meetings reassuring and motivating. Others find them distasteful. Some patients come just a few times shortly after their surgery. Others become active for the long term, often volunteering their support to new patients. If your hospital has a support group, consider going. If nothing else, you will make contact with others who have walked your path, and they may be able to answer your questions. This peer group can be especially valuable if you have little questions you have not been able to discuss with your doctor. If your hospital does not have a support group, look to the American Heart Association for a nearby chapter of Mended Hearts, the support group AHA has sponsored for thirty years. To locate Mended Hearts, call your local American Heart Association office or the national headquarters in Dallas at (214) 373-6300.

## Managing Insistent Problems

While most patients experience satisfactory progress in the weeks following discharge, persistent complaints send a small proportion of patients back to their cardiologists. Usually, physicians can solve the problem, but occasionally they shrug their shoulders and say, "There's nothing wrong." Actually, they mean they can't find anything wrong. Put another way, they mean that if there were something seriously wrong, they would most likely spot it; since they don't see it, it is probably not a threatening problem, bothersome and worrisome though it might feel.

Like everyone else, physicians prefer to be effective, and not being able to resolve their patients' medical complaints can make them uncomfortable. As a result, they may retreat. If you sense your physician is avoiding you, you may feel neglected, become angry, and perhaps depressed. If you find yourself with this problem, consider discussing it with a psychological counselor, who may be able to help you devise a strategy for solving it.

You might also consider asking your physician for a consultation with another cardiologist. In perplexing cases, a second opinion may provide valuable insight. At the very least, it can reassure you and your cardiologist that your treatment has been appropriate. Most doctors welcome the request for a second opinion, and you should not be embarrassed to ask for one.

## Making Major Changes

Experts recommend making as few major changes in your life as possible for a year following surgery, and for good reason. Many patients have acknowledged that their surgery skewed their perspectives temporarily. Soon after surgery, they thought they wanted to retire or move to a new city or get married or get divorced. But a year or so later, they discovered they had made a mistake. In addition, when people move to a new city, leave their familiar workplace, or make a similarly major change, they often cut down their support systems just when they need them most. Finally, major life changes require people to strain their coping reserves; because of heart surgery, those coping reserves have already been strained. Overtaxing them might invite depression.

## Returning to Work

You will probably get permission to return to work within two months after surgery. Though you are returning to work, you will still get tired. Don't be surprised if you feel more tired than you have for weeks—just as you may have felt you had regressed when you left the ICU and then again when you left the hospital. Increased challenges are likely to exaggerate your vulnerability. Test your strength; make time to rest; save time to exercise;

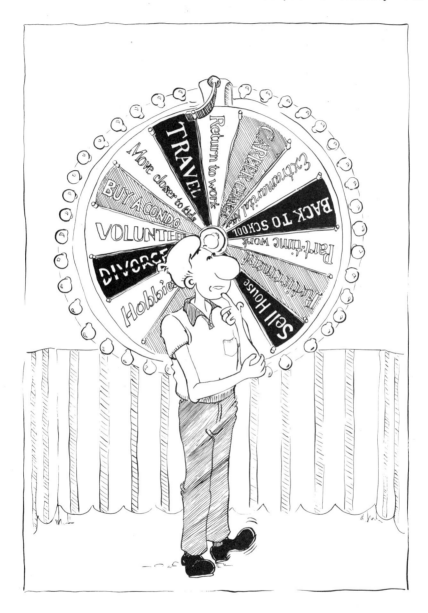

Experts recommend making as few major changes in your life as possible for a year following surgery.

don't be impatient. Remember, many patients need a full year to overcome all the lingering effects of their surgery.

After bypass surgery, some patients elect to take a demotion, together with a pay cut, in order to reduce their stress. Most patients can return to their former employment. And many patients who had been disabled are suddenly well enough to work again. They return to jobs as mechanics, truck drivers, plumbers, and electricians, as well as to numerous office positions.

You will, of course, return to work with your doctor's approval, probably even a formal letter attesting to your well-being. Don't be surprised, however, if you experience discrimination at work. Some employers read "bypass" on an employment report and see the red flag of absenteeism and increased insurance costs. Others refuse newly returning workers any consideration or leeway whatsoever. Still others behave as though bypass is somehow catching and attempt to ostracize newly returning workers.

Sad to say, many patients have had unsavory experiences in this regard. A truck driver was told he had to resume all his responsibilities four weeks after surgery or lose his job. A counselor from Mended Hearts intervened on his behalf, and the patient was given a desk job temporarily. In a separate instance, a mechanic for a major airline was told to remain on leave until he was able to return full time and perform all his duties. Fortunately, this man's co-workers pitched in to help with his heaviest work until he could lift sixty pounds or more. A third patient, with a long and excellent record as a factory foreman, experienced serious discrimination when he moved to a new city and tried to get a job. Seven times he applied, and seven times, mysteriously, he got no job. On the eighth try, by coincidence, he encountered a different interviewer, who sent him to the company physician for a physical immediately.

"Usually you get your physical after you're hired. In my case, they changed the procedure, so I knew they were discriminating. But when the company doc sent back a report that said I was in better shape then he was, they hired me," he reported.

Ideally, you'll have no such trouble. But if you do, you don't have to sit by and accept it. Perhaps your union or the social service department of your hospital can intervene on your behalf. If necessary, contact the American Civil Liberties Union, a private attorney, the federally funded legal services office nearest you, or a local office of the Equal Employment Opportunity Commission.

In addition, most experts—professionals as well as former patients—would advise against changing jobs at this time. There is the danger of potential discrimination as well as the added stress the change would create. If, when you return to work, you find yourself in a less desirable job because your old position was filled in your absence, don't quit precipitously. Consider your options carefully. If you must change jobs, you would do well to seek career counseling and get some good advice on how to handle your medical history when you apply for a new job.

Executive career counselor Diane Railton, president of Taylor Mark Stanley and Company, recommends withholding the information during the application and interview process as long as possible. If you are asked, you must answer truthfully because, she feels, there is nothing more damaging than lying. If no one asks, however, she advises that you say nothing until you are offered the job. At that point, say something like, "There's something in my medical history I feel I should tell you. I had bypass surgery four months ago, but I'm fine now. Of course, I'll give you a letter from my physician to confirm that, and I'll be happy to submit to whatever physical exam you require." Diane Railton feels that the majority of employers she deals with would not reject a candidate on the basis of bypass.

Contact the social service department of your hospital or a career counselor for further guidance.

## Points to Remember

❏ At first, stay alone for only a short time.

❏ Alternate activities and rest.

❏ Anticipate fatigue, and increase exercise gradually.

❏ Begin massaging the chest incision during the third week.

❏ Continue breathing exercises through the fourth week.

❏ Try a bed-time ritual to cure insomnia.

❏ Approach a low-fat diet with a sense of adventure.

❏ Be patient and candid as you resume sex.

❏ Take advantage of peer support groups to share experiences and resolve concerns.

❏ Avoid making major changes for a year.

Chapter Eight

# WHEN SOMEONE YOU LOVE HAS HEART SURGERY

As difficult as heart surgery can be, many patients contend that it is more difficult on the people who love them than on the patients themselves. Unwittingly, patients often reveal why.

## Stresses Inherent in the Role of Supporter

Stuart McConnell reported, "The night before surgery, Helen cried and said she was worried I would die. 'I'm not going to die,' I said, 'but if I do, it doesn't matter because I'll be dead and I won't care.'"

Like many spouses and other primary supporters, Helen McConnell saw her husband's heart condition and his surgery as a threat to herself and her future, and she chastised herself for such selfish feelings. In the ensuing weeks, worry, guilt, and depression ate away at her.

The evening before surgery, while her husband managed his anxiety by asking the anesthesiologist, surgeon, respiratory therapist, physical therapist, and clinical nurse specialist a long list of questions, Mrs. McConnell went home to an empty house.

"I tried to read, but I couldn't concentrate. I turned on the television, but it hammered at my head. Finally, at midnight, I got into bed, but my heart was pounding and my mind was racing. I was whipped, but there was no sleep for me that night."

Meanwhile, Stuart McConnell took a sedative, which put him and his anxieties to rest.

Throughout her husband's hospitalization, Mrs. McConnell maintained her full-time job as a bookkeeper,

153

did her husband's household chores as well as her own, and visited her husband after work every evening. She grew increasingly exhausted, felt her fears erupt every time his progress seemed to slow, and tried to marshal all her patience to cope with his periodic irritability. Once he got home, she felt responsible for his welfare. Afraid that he would overexert himself or suffer a setback, she hovered over him relentlessly. She reached to pour him a glass of juice and jumped up to the door when the bell rang. She nagged at him to rest, and she nagged at him to exercise. As he exploded, "Get the hell off my back," she felt her anger and resentment boil.

"The primary supporters have a tremendous burden," asserted counselor Sally Kolitz. "They share all the patient's worries. Plus they have extra work. They get exhausted. They often experience verbal and emotional assault. But the system is not designed to give them support. Usually, that's reserved for the patient, but those who love him need it every bit as much."

## The Value of Supporters

Your role as a supporter is a vital one. Many patients have attributed the speed and ease of their recovery to good marriages, devoted children, and caring friends. Medical professionals observe that having someone to get well for often motivates patients to recover. One patient, who became demoralized when he developed a wound infection and clots in his lungs, claimed his dedication to his family sustained him through three weeks of hospitalization. Though he was discouraged, he insisted, "I won't give up. I can't chuck it because of my boys."

Undoubtedly, this patient's commitment to his sons enhanced his will to recover, and when he was finally discharged, he anticipated an uncompromised recovery.

Numerous studies confirm the importance of social support. You can offer valuable insights, information, and fresh ideas for solving problems. You can also provide material aid, understanding, and distractions from discomfort. With proper skill and sensitivity, you can ease your loved one's crisis tremendously, and your relationship can grow stronger and healthier than it was before. To provide support effectively, however, you need to take care of yourself as well as the patient you love.

## Acquiring Information

Just as patients benefit from information designed to help them cope with the bypass experience, so you can benefit from knowledge as well. You might want to attend patient education classes and introductory sessions with the various therapists. At the same time, be sure to respect the patient's right, as well as your own, to have some private time with the medical personnel for confidential discussions. If you can strike a comfortable balance between protecting individual privacy and participating constructively in the presurgical consultations, you can set the scene for mutual respect and understanding.

In addition to learning about surgery and recovery, it's a good idea to get the following information for yourself:

*Where can I wait during surgery?*

*What kind of progress reports can I expect and how long will I have to wait for the first one?* (Some hospitals are wonderfully considerate of the anxiety families feel from the moment they kiss their patients good luck. And while these hospitals are good about providing progress reports, the first one often comes when the heart-lung machine takes over the patient's cardiac and respiratory functions, sometimes as long as two hours into surgery.)

*Who will deliver these reports?*

*When can I speak to the doctor?*

*When can I first see my patient following surgery, and what will he or she look like? What kinds of tubes, catheters, wires, and machinery can I expect to encounter? Will the patient be sleeping or awake? Coherent or foggy? Will his complexion look healthy or wan? Will I see blood?* (The answers to these questions depend, in part, on how soon after surgery visitors are allowed into the ICU.)

*What are the visiting hours in the ICU? If I feel concerned between visiting hours, whom can I call?*

Keep pencil and paper handy to note questions, jot down key points, and list additional questions. Answers to the first questions always provoke new ones, and in the stress of the moment, unless you write them down, you may forget them.

After the patient-orientation session, many supporters and patients find it helpful to review together what they learned and questions they still have. Sometimes supporters and patients interpret information differently and remember different points. Going over the information clarifies the truth and creates an opportunity to share feelings. Honest talk can clear the air and bring people closer together, provided each person respects the other's coping preferences and need for privacy.

## Conflicting Coping Styles

One husband who attended all his wife's surgical education sessions found the experience upsetting. Though the patient eagerly sought every possible detail, her husband found that each new bit of knowledge made him worry more. He would have done better to wait outside.

Another supporter encountered difficulty when she sensed her husband didn't share her need to talk about his forthcoming surgery. "I had a very tough time before my husband's surgery. My husband is very independent. He had to go into the hospital himself, get all his information himself, and when I came to visit him, he insisted on talking about anything but his operation. It was so frustrating for me, I left his room in tears."

To cope with impending surgery, this patient had to demonstrate to himself that he was invincible. He always handled problems in his life alone, and this one would be no exception. His wife needed to talk through her fears, but she realized that it would be wrong to impose her anxieties on her husband. Fortunately, she encountered the patient education specialist, who lent her an untiring ear. This sensitive nurse listened to all her fears, answered all her questions, and promised to see her in the surgical waiting room the next morning.

If your coping styles differ from your patient's, you must defer to his. But you must meet your own needs as well. If you need to talk, find someone else to talk to. By taking care of yourself, you will improve your capacity to be a good supporter later.

# Empathy

Tuning in to the kind of support that is genuinely helpful to another person—a child, a lover, a friend, a patient—means being a compassionate listener. It involves the skills psychologists include when they talk about empathy or active listening. For patients coping with heart surgery this is the most important service any loved one can provide.

When you listen compassionately, you experience another person's feelings as if they were your own. You make no judgments about what the other person is feeling. You simply try to understand it. In so doing, you acknowledge that you respect the other person. At the same time, you refrain from implying that any emotional response is better or worse than any other.

As Sylvia Turner bent over to kiss her husband goodnight the evening before his surgery, he addressed the emotions that held his body rigid. "I'm so terrified of tomorrow," he whispered. "I'm afraid I'll never kiss you good-night again."

"Of course you're terrified," Sylvia Turner replied. "Anyone going into heart surgery could be frightened. But remember that the doctor said you're an excellent candidate. It's o.k. to be scared, but you will do fine. You're going to come through this operation like a champ."

Sylvia Turner accepted her husband's apprehension and acknowledged its legitimacy. She also reminded him that, while his fears were understandable, there were many reasons to be optimistic. That's very different from saying his fears were wrong.

Too many spouses, themselves feeling threatened by the experience or the emotions it evokes, might respond, "Don't worry. Everything will be all right." That's what Anita Brown did.

Never, to Anita Brown's recollection, had her husband faltered in his strength. He built a brilliant business, and he made all financial and practical decisions for his family. Now seventy-six and retired, he continued to portray confidence and independence, and Anita Brown admitted that, after fifty-two years of marriage, she leaned on her husband shamelessly. Imagine the scene when, on the sixth day after Gerald Brown's surgery, Anita Brown walked into her husband's room and found him sobbing like a little boy.

"He was terrified that he had lost his mind, and I was terrified that I was losing him," Anita Brown remembered. "You know, before the operation he said everything would be fine, and I believed him. I was worried, sure, but I never really believed he would die. When I saw him in the intensive care unit, he didn't look so good, but I knew it was temporary. But when I saw him crying, that was too much. He shouldn't know I'm upset, I thought, so I said, 'Gerry, don't cry. You're gonna be fine. There's nothing to worry about. Remember, Joey's coming from California to see you tonight.'"

Anita Brown hoped that her platitudes would dry her husband's tears and bring the smile of self-confidence back into his eyes. Perhaps making these statements helped her deny that her husband was not the emotional Samson she wished him to be. But they did not resolve Gerald Brown's own fears about his physical and emotional weakness, nor did they erase the feelings that caused his tears in the first place. By offering banalities and implying that she did not understand what he was feeling, Anita Brown alienated herself from her husband. She might have helped her husband while strengthening the bond between them if she had empathized with his misery.

"It's o.k. to cry," she might have said. "There's nothing wrong with crying when you're fed up with being sick. I understand your frustration, and maybe crying will help a little."

In the day or so before surgery, empathy can take the form of acknowledging fear or respecting denial. In the days, weeks, and months afterwards, it can shift to understanding anxiety, fear, and anger. Empathy can open the door to solving real problems:

*I appreciate your frustration at not being able to talk to the doctor. Perhaps we can ask him to allow ten extra minutes tomorrow.*

*Of course you're entitled to feel blue. Listening to Bill Cosby always used to perk you up. What do you think about getting a Cosby tape from the library?*

*I would be short-tempered, too, if I got tired just from reading the morning newspaper. But we need to find a way not to take out our frustrations on each other.*

Empathy suggests, "She really does understand," and while understanding doesn't eradicate the problem, it's a good beginning.

Whether patients acknowledge fear going into surgery or not, most are affected by it at least on an unconscious level. While candor is important, destroying a person's defenses can be devastating, and a supporter who tries to drag an admission of fear from a patient who seems at peace can wreck the patient's self-protective mechanisms. As the moments before surgery draw closer, take your cues from your loved one. And as you kiss him good luck, you would do well to imply that survival and recovery are certain. A statement like "I'll see you when you wake up" can do wonders to lower anxiety.

## Coping with the ICU

You usually can visit the ICU briefly within an hour or so after surgery. It takes this long for patients to be settled and hooked up to their various machines and monitors. When you see your loved one for the first time, he will probably still be anesthetized and lying utterly still. He may have surprisingly pink color. He is likely to be covered up to his chin, so you won't see the myriad tubes and catheters which have been plugged into his body. What you will see is the endotracheal tube, which is taped to the face and connected to the respirator, and the naso-gastric tube, which emerges from the nose and is also taped in place.

"When the counselor invited me into the ICU for the first time, I felt bombarded by mixed emotions," the husband of a bypass patient recalled. "I was relieved, of course, because the counselor assured me my wife was o.k. But I felt really skittish about seeing her in that condition. Everything I had heard about the ICU spooked me, and I followed that counselor in dread."

This is a common moment for tears.

"It's relief," assessed Barbara Friedman. "They've spent all this energy worrying. And they're exhausted. Once they see with their own eyes that everything is as it should be, they let go. After a quick peek to reassure themselves, I urge our patients' families to go home, have a cup of tea, and get some rest."

## Being Supportive in the ICU

In retrospect, former patients feel a number of items would have made their time in ICU easier. Before visiting in the ICU, you might put together a help package based on these suggestions. If your patient wears glasses, bring an extra pair in case the pair he was wearing before surgery didn't find its way to the ICU. To help an intubated patient communicate, bring a large clipboard with plenty of big sheets of paper and a short, fat pencil. These are the easiest implements to use for a patient whose arm is strapped to an IV board. Since nurses step away from the bedside momentarily, bring something an intubated patient can use to attract attention. A large paper fastener or a hemostat—a medical instrument that looks like a cross between eyebrow tweezers and a pair of scissors—is ideal because you can clip it to the bed sheet and bang it against the bedrail. Sometimes patients also appreciate having a clock and a Walkman-type radio. Before bringing in these last two items, however, you would be wise to look over the ICU setup, assess the appropriateness of the idea, and mention it to the nurses. Often patients are in ICU so briefly and the quarters are so cramped that bringing in this kind of equipment would create more problems than it would solve.

If you are visiting when your patient rouses from anesthesia, you can contribute significantly to reorienting him. Since general anesthesia always disorients patients, they benefit tremendously from hearing, "You're fine, Dad. Your surgery is over and everything is o.k." Telling him what day and time it is also helps. Patients characteristically drift into and out of awareness for several hours and often need these messages repeated.

Though visits in the ICU are short, you can fulfill a vital role during this difficult period. While your patient is intubated, help him communicate non-verbally by calmly and quietly attempting to understand his message. In the event of difficulty, do not ask him questions he cannot answer. Talk calmly and quietly. Reassure him that you will figure out what he wants even if it takes some time. Pat his arms. Soothe him verbally. Devise a progression of yes-no questions which he can answer by moving his head or blinking his eyes.

Encourage him to lie quietly and permit the medical staff to take care of him. Encourage him to trust the medical personnel.

If he remains disoriented after the intubation tube is removed and if he is aware he is not himself, urge him to talk about his fears. Pat his head, stroke his forehead, caress his cheek; touching provides additional reassurance.

You can also help by reaffirming that he is entitled not to like the medical treatments that are imposed on him and that he would be justified in feeling angry at the nurses and therapists whose treatments feel like torture. If you say something like, "It's normal for people to feel irritable when they hurt," or "You don't have to like your treatments; you just have to take them," you will validate his anger and help him to realize that the nurses understand it and don't take it personally. Tufts University professor of psychiatry Richard Blacher discovered that when patients believe that their anger will not alienate their caretakers, they are less likely to encounter serious emotional distress.

Above all, in the unlikely event that your patient makes irrational claims, do not argue with him or attempt to convince him that his perceptions are wrong.

One patient in the ICU was terribly agitated because he was convinced something was wrong with his IV. Before long, the patient's growing distress had drawn two nurses and a physician's assistant to his bedside. Foolishly, these three professionals argued louder and louder that his IV was fine.

At that moment, the patient's daughter came to the bedside and took over management of the problem.

"Dad, I think there's something wrong with your IV, but I can't figure out what it is. Will you please help me and I'll see that it's fixed," she said.

In the stupor of his medications, the patient didn't convey his ideas too clearly, but with patience and persistence, the daughter was able to discern that he was distressed because the IV tube was twisted and he was afraid the fluids could not flow freely.

"Do you think it would help if we shortened the IV tube so that it couldn't twist?" she asked.

He heaved a thankful yes. The nurse took a link out of the IV tubing, and the patient relaxed.

When patients respond irrationally, do not try to convince them they are wrong. First, it doesn't work. And second, since their disorientation is temporary, it doesn't matter. What does matter is that their anxiety is put to rest. That can be accomplished by assuming the problem, as they perceive it, is valid and attempting to solve it.

# Being Supportive for the Duration of Recovery

Once your patient moves into step-down care and throughout the recuperative period at home, your role changes. Now, rather than soothing and calming him, you must direct your energies to reinforcing the self-help messages of the medical personnel.

"I know it hurts to cough, but you have to do it. I know you're tired, but you have to walk" is the theme.

You can also help by restoring the patient's sense of control as much as possible and by attempting to make him feel whole, needed, and important. Ask your patient for his opinion, seek his advice, and offer him choices. Permit him his anger and fears, and share yours. Resist the inclination to protect him from problems.

## Anxiety and Its Consequences

Too often, the supporters' worries get in their way. Feeling threatened, they often make inappropriately optimistic remarks. When they cannot acknowledge their fears and those of the patient they love, they sometimes erect a wall of isolation. And when patients sense that their families cannot handle their illness, they feel abandoned.

One supporter, terrified that her husband would never work again, could not face his anxieties over the same thought. A construction foreman whose angina had kept him from work for six months, he was obsessed about what kind of job he could hold after his recovery. His wife was aware of his concerns, but she could not bear to discuss them. Whenever possible, she changed the subject. When pressed, she ignored its significance.

"What are you thinking about that now for? You're still in the hospital. Worry about getting home first," she advised, wedging an uncomfortable distance between them.

Another wife, afraid to agitate her husband, stopped consulting him as problems arose concerning the country home they were building. Whereas before surgery they talked to the contractor together, after his surgery she shielded him from such talks. While he was in the hospital, she lied that she hadn't been in touch with the contractor. After he came home, she pretended someone else called on the phone.

"One time, the contractor called to say the plumbing fixtures hadn't been delivered. Another time, he said he had to put the electrician on another job for a week. Delays like this drive my husband crazy, and I know stress is bad for him," Patricia Teller explained.

While Patricia Teller meant well, she angered her husband and strained their relationship. She worried silently about distressing him, and he quietly seethed that he was not as vulnerable as she presumed. Instead of sharing their feelings about his health and their retirement home, each tried to cope separately. They stopped relating, and they stopped communicating.

To be sure, Patricia Teller's behavior was prompted by concern for Robert Teller's welfare. At home, separated from constant medical supervision, she feared stress would trigger a setback. She was unclear about exactly what activities or emotional involvements constituted stress, so she attempted to prevent them all.

Patricia Teller's errors are common. Many supporters are uncertain about how their patients should be feeling from day to day, and exactly what activities and involvements are safe. Out of fear and uncertainty, they smother their patients, and the patients become less independent and more sedentary than they had been in the hospital.

When patients have a bad day—as they all do—their supporters hover even more closely. To break the cycle, patients often hide their discomforts, thus increasing the distance between the parties.

In truth, Robert Teller was more frustrated by his wife's overprotection than he would have been by the construction delays. If he had been informed, he would have felt a sense of participation, and that feeling would have tempered his frustrations.

Of course, everyone is different, and sometimes patients find an element of comfort in overprotection.

"I was grateful for my wife's vigilance," said one such patient. "I liked knowing she was concerned. She was there all the time, watching me. She'd wake up in the middle of the night to make sure I was breathing, and I knew that if anything happened, she'd see that I got help."

In most instances, however, patients find that hovering supporters emphasize unpleasant feelings of insecurity and unworthiness. If patients already view themselves as damaged goods and worry that others view them similarly, reminders of their fragility can infuriate them. Their anger can then alienate family and friends, and a bad situation gets worse.

One former patient recalled the frustration he felt as almost everyone he knew made a special effort to take care of him. "It was as though I was living in a padded world. Even months after my surgery, when the doctor had given me the green light to do everything, my secretary jumped up to take my briefcase when I came in to work in the morning. My tennis partner didn't hit as close to the lines as he used to. My buddies wouldn't even get into a good debate over politics anymore. Everybody treated me as though they were afraid I would break, and I hated it."

If overprotection is a problem, the solution is probably increased knowledge. When you and your loved one are confident that recovery is progressing properly, when you are convinced that certain activities and involvements are therapeutic, and when you feel you can distinguish between signs of trouble and benign symptoms, you will probably be able to relax. Therefore, you need to keep asking questions until you have concrete and satisfactory answers. Knowing vaguely that a patient should "do a little more but continue taking it easy" isn't good enough. How far should he be walking this week? How many hours can she work? Which responsibilities can she assume? In what way is healing pain different from heart pain? When you get satisfying answers to questions like these, you will probably be able to provide constructive support to your patient. As the two of you share your concerns and reassure each other, you're likely to strengthen the bond between you.

## Feeling Overwhelmed

The stresses that you experience during this period can wear you down. Often, supporters let their hectic schedules, their worries, and their dedication drive them to exhaustion. As one wife admitted, "While my husband was in the hospital, I ran on nervous energy. I was at the hospital before eight every morning to help him with breakfast, and I stayed until after dinner because he was too weak to feed himself. By the time he came home, I was a little run down."

Another supporter agreed. "The driving back and forth was hard. Anxiety made it worse. And once I got home at night, the incessant phone calls drove me to distraction. People meant well, but I couldn't deal with it anymore. In desperation, I put a nightly progress report on my answering machine and turned the ringer off."

Whether the supporters are men or women, they are invariably faced with new challenges which, in light of the surrounding stresses, become more difficult than they would otherwise be. When their husbands are hospitalized, many women confront their first experiences with

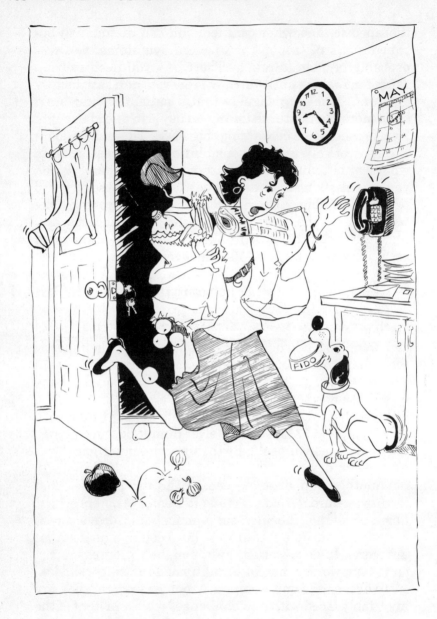

Often, supporters let their hectic schedules, their worries, and their dedication drive them to exhaustion.

bank accounts and insurance policies. Occasionally, when continuing medical problems or job discrimination forces their husbands to retire, women face working outside the home for the first time in many years. When the patients are women, many men experience the alien role of nurturer. Some have no idea about how to do the laundry, feel helpless in the kitchen or the supermarket, and quake at the prospect of being responsible for their wives' welfare.

"We had been married forty years, but when my wife came home from the hospital, I didn't know what to say to her or what to do for her. My hands would shake if I had to give her her medicine," one husband admitted.

Unmarried patients present other difficulties for supporters. Often children or siblings must leave their families and travel to another city to care for a recuperating patient. Divided loyalties and conflicting responsibilities invariably add to their concerns.

Even when someone feels comfortable as a primary supporter, heart surgery can exaggerate the inherent difficulties in the role. A wife admitted, "Between worrying about my job, his well-being, and my crazy schedule, I got lost in the woods of worry. I couldn't figure out which ones were important and which were trivial. I needed help sorting out what to focus on and what to forget."

## Guilt and Resentment

Sometimes feelings of guilt and responsibility surface. One wife, whose husband was taking iron tablets to cure his postoperative anemia, served liver his first night home because she knew it was rich in iron.

"After dinner, he got pain in his chest and needed a nitroglycerine, and I was sure I had caused the problem," she recalled.

When patients understand the strains their supporters feel, the patients can do a lot to ease them. Sometimes, however, patients are so preoccupied with their own problems that they become oblivious to anyone else's. One former patient, proud of the superwoman who was his wife, breezily dismissed questions about her difficulties by saying, "She rose to the occasion."

In addition, patients' irritability, a common sequel to surgery, eats away at their supporters' capacity to cope. In the weeks following surgery, some patients become demanding and difficult to please. Supporters occasionally find themselves turning their own lives inside out to care for someone whose personality they hardly recognize. The slower the patient's recovery and the lower the levels of empathy and communication, the more intense these problems become.

One patient, seriously depressed but unwilling to face his depression, turned away from his family entirely. Months after his surgery, he seemed a different person. Whereas he had always been involved with his family and their activities, he suddenly disappeared for days at a time. When he was home, he was sullen and remote. Understandably, his wife was devastated.

"I had worked so hard to be supportive and take care of him," she complained. "He never acknowledged the toll his illness took on me. And then he just shut me out. Always before we talked through dinner and long into the night. And now we don't talk at all."

This example represents the extreme. More often the changes are less dramatic.

"There were no big issues, but the little issues never quit," one wife commented. "He wanted a turkey sandwich for lunch, and as soon as I made it, he asked for tuna. I tried so hard to please him, but it seemed I couldn't do anything right."

Typically, patients vent their anger at their supporters, the people they care about most. Unconsciously, they realize that these people, whose love they can rely on, make safe targets. While the anger is, in a perverse fashion, a statement of trust, it is not easy to take. The supporters, who have dedicated themselves to caretaking, lose their patience under the barrage of irritability. Supporters also feel guilty because of their resentment and to some degree because they are healthy. Paradoxically, while supporters initially feel overwhelmed by too many concerns, after the patient is home for a short time, their focus grows uncomfortably narrow.

"Before I realized it, I had no life of my own. I was with my husband constantly. I served him. I walked with him. I tried new recipes for him. I drove him to cardiac rehab. In the process, I stopped my volunteer work. I never had lunch with my friends. I never thought about anything unrelated to heart disease," one supporter said.

Another supporter agreed. "I'm so tired of thinking about illness. My husband is so self-centered. He's preoccupied with his food and his rest and his exercise. He says he needs to be in order to get well and stay well. But he won't give up demanding the attention that goes with being sick."

If these problems weren't enough, they become aggravated when, in a well-intentioned attempt to support the patient, friends and extended family overlook the supporters' own need for help.

## Resolving the Problems

Fortunately, these difficulties usually resolve themselves within a few months after surgery. As patients grow stronger and healthier, their anger and depression abate. They resume their old lifestyle or adjust to a new one, they lose their preoccupation with themselves, and their former personalities reemerge. During the crisis, however, you need to protect yourself.

Self-protection begins when you relinquish feelings of responsibility for your loved one's recovery. If your patient does not recuperate quickly or refuses to take responsibility for his recovery, don't get trapped into feeling you have failed. You did not make your loved one sick, and you cannot fix his troubles. Ultimately, the responsibility for doing the work of recovery lies with the patient.

In addition to freeing yourself from this impossible responsibility, you must make sure that you take care of yourself. Many people who have traveled this road recommend asking for help. Friends, neighbors, and relatives appreciate feeling needed and often welcome specific requests. "Please cook dinner tonight. Please take the clothes to the cleaners or stop at the supermarket or stay with Fred on Friday afternoon."

Communicate your feelings with your patient and solicit his support for you. One wife's experience dramatizes how effective this approach can be. Although her husband was recuperating well, she found herself growing increasingly exhausted and resentful. As she walked in from work one night, she burst into tears.

"Honey, what's wrong?" her startled husband asked.

"I'm so tired of going to work and taking care of this house and taking care of you. I know it's not your fault that you got sick, but I can't help the way I feel," she cried.

"What can I do to help you?" her husband asked.

After thinking a minute, she responded, "If you'd just do the breakfast dishes so I didn't have to walk into a dirty kitchen when I come home from work, I think it would help."

The next morning, her husband not only did the dishes, but scrubbed the counters, shined the stove top, and polished the refrigerator. He was delighted to be doing something that mattered. When his wife came home that evening, she felt a rush of appreciation and partnership instead of the familiar resentment. By telling her husband what she needed, she, as well as her husband, got more than just a clean kitchen.

If giving health care seems overbearing, call the Visiting Nurse's Association or the American Heart Association for supportive health services. If finances perplex you, ask an officer at the bank to help demystify Certificates of Deposit and checkbooks; she is paid to offer such assistance. If possible, hire a maid for a few hours a week or take the laundry to a wash and fold.

Most important, set aside time for yourself. This is not time taken away from the patient; it is time to replenish your own resources so that you can be a better caretaker. Unburden yourself by confiding in an empathic friend. Talk to others who have been in your position, and get reassurance that this difficult period will end. Make arrangements to keep up with your weekly bridge game or go out to lunch with a friend or meet your stockbroker or take a bubble bath. Invariably, professionals agree, if you can compensate for your stresses and restore facets of your normal life, you will speed the crisis of illness to an end. If you cannot reduce your stress with efforts like these, seek crisis intervention counseling for yourself. A professional can probably view your problems with enough perspective to help you devise effective solutions.

Ultimately, the crisis will be over. Rarely is it resolved leaving the participants the same as they had been before.

"The experience is too profound for people to walk away from it untouched," believes Sally Kolitz. "One way or another, patients and their supporters are bound to be different afterwards."

Occasionally, as patients grow stronger and reclaim their former roles, their supporters have trouble because they feel they are no longer needed. Conversely, recuperating patients may feel reluctant to relinquish the sick role even though, by all medical measures, they should be functioning as well people. Difficulties like these as well as less clear-cut problems, especially among couples whose marriages were shaky before the surgery, sometimes result in permanently impaired relationships. At least as frequently, however, families and friendships emerge stronger and closer for having come through the crisis together.

On a practical level, supporters discover they have capabilities they never would have imagined possible. One wife realized how vulnerable she was being ignorant about finances. After her husband's recuperation, she became expert not only at paying bills and balancing the checkbook but at understanding insurance policies and managing investments. Whether supporters take on new roles permanently or resort to old ones, many emerge from the experience feeling more independent and self-reliant. Others discover the powerful bonding crises can promote.

"When my father had bypass, I came from New York and my sister came from Denver, and for the first time in years we had something more important to say to each other than 'What's new?'" one adult child observed. "Our whole family is closer as a result."

Similarly, many marriages have benefited. Partners commonly claim the experience made them appreciate each other more, understand each other better, and place new value on the times they shared.

One former patient summed up the impact of the crisis this way: "It's so easy to take a marriage for granted. When my husband realized that I could die and I realized how much I needed him, we were shaken out of our complacency. Life and love are so fragile. Now we devote a lot of time to protecting them."

# Points to Remember

❑ Satisfy your own needs to acquire information and resolve concerns.

❑ Try to listen to your patient and accept his feelings without being judgmental.

❑ Be reassuring and comforting in the ICU.

❑ Encourage independence later.

❏ Avoid being overprotective.

❏ Take care of yourself.

❏ Seek help and social support when you need it.

❏ Try to restore facets of your normal life as quickly as possible.

## Chapter Nine

# MORE ABOUT DEPRESSION

To a great extent, depression after heart surgery is a normal response. The antithesis to the stress and anxiety of the immediate pre- and postoperative periods, it is the mind's retreat, a hide-away for repair and restoration.

As the preceding chapters revealed, depression occasionally descends while patients are in the ICU, but it usually waits until after they test their strength in a regular hospital room. This is when they discover how weak they are and begin to question the effectiveness of their surgery. In their weakened condition, they tend to perceive small difficulties as major problems. As they struggle, their families tend to coddle them, and they feel worse. Going home sets patients up for a recurrence of these feelings. Most patients ready for discharge have overcome the fatigue they felt during the early days in a regular hospital room, and by the time they are discharged, they feel fine. Then the trip home exhausts them, and the pattern repeats. To aggravate it, the limits of recuperation seem more exaggerated at home than they did in the protective environment of the hospital, and patients sometimes conclude the road to recovery is more tortuous than they had thought. Normal reactive depression results. It can come and go for as long as three months. Usually, the bad days grow more distant from one another, and then they disappear.

## Reactive Depression and Grief

The depression that patients normally experience after surgery strongly resembles the grief that survivors, particularly spouses, feel when a loved one dies. Peggy Eastman, contributing editor for *Self* magazine, described her feelings of despair after her husband had been killed in an airplane crash. Her appetite disappeared. Sleep became an elusive friend to be lured, but only briefly, by sedatives. Panic, like a stalking cat, caught her off guard. It attacked unprovoked with startling surprise, and smothered perspective and reason before succumbing to a Xanax[†] pill. Worse, it made her feel "freakish, distanced, set apart. . . . I was a pariah, as if I had done something embarrassing, something that made people around me feel uncomfortable. What people seemed to want was for me to be 'recovered,' returned as quickly as possible to the person they knew before. But I couldn't do it."

Like grief, the depression which follows surgery has a specific reason. Like grief, it is painful but usually not dangerous. It mimics clinical depression, which is a chronic illness that often demands active and prolonged medical treatment. But unlike more menacing depressions, it is usually self-limiting. Within several months it should go away. In addition—and this is important— normal reactive depression rarely causes long-term feelings of worthlessness and guilt.

## The Many Faces of Depression

For all this seemingly clear-cut description, reactive depression can present a muddy multitude of portraits, some diametrically different from others. While some of the pictures are benign, others are pernicious. And the line between them, characterized largely by the severity and duration of symptoms, is easily blurred. Because the signs can be so ambiguous, lingering depression can go un- diagnosed and untreated. Yet in its most severe forms it can impose such heavy feelings of hopelessness that vic- tims contemplate suicide. This is rare. However, since reactive depression does, on occasion, become danger- ously severe, we will try to resolve the ambiguity.

[†] Upjohn (Alprazolan)

In its most benign form, depression seems no different from the transient pessimism and disinterest most people experience briefly when the weather turns gloomy or work gets boring. While it feels heavy, the weight is not unbearable and it lifts readily. In its more debilitating forms, depression can make independent adults regress into a dependent, childlike state. It can make people who, by all medical measures, should feel strong and healthy feel sick and weak, sometimes for years on end.

"It was the darkest, most terrifying and painful period of my life," said one patient who first encountered depression following his coronary bypass surgery. "It was more frightening than being in the Normandy Invasion, more painful than losing my wife, and worse than any other illness I've ever had."

Like people suffering from less serious forms, those who experience worrisome depression usually—but not always—feel sad, discouraged, or hopeless. In addition, they often lose interest in activities which ordinarily stimulate them and find that nothing brings them pleasure. They may lose their drive and their persistence, saying they just don't care. While depression is almost always associated with some of these feelings, some victims withdraw rather than complain. Refusing to see family and friends, they may spend hours lying listlessly in bed or sitting in a darkened room. And sometimes, depression, especially after surgery, is marked solely by feeling physically sick.

Those who are depressed often complain that they cannot concentrate. Sometimes their thinking slows down; their memory fails, and they find themselves easily distracted. Yet they often brood and become obsessed about their physical health. They may become phobic or suddenly panic. Frequently they look gloomy and feel anxious. They may cry for no apparent reason. Pernicious depression often makes people suffer low self-esteem. Ridden by a sense of guilt and worthlessness, they often

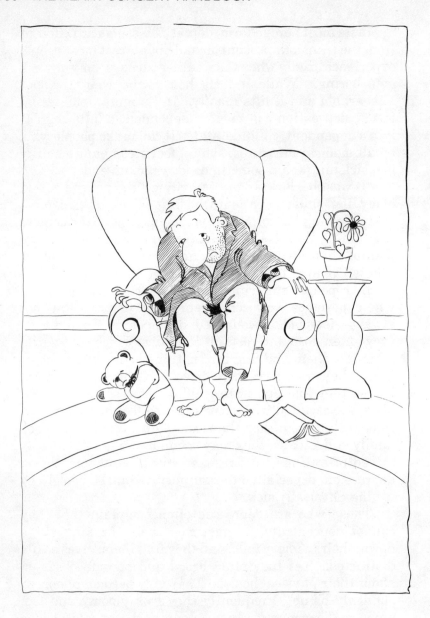

Refusing to see family and friends, they may spend hours lying listlessly in bed or sitting in a darkened room.

feel responsible for events beyond their control. At worst, they may hallucinate, become obsessed about some presumed sinfulness or worthlessness, or worry that they will succumb to illness, poverty, or some vague source of destruction. With these feelings may come a fear of dying, thoughts of suicide, or death wishes.

"Everyone would be better off if I were dead" is a frequent lament.

In addition, victims of depression may experience a change in eating habits. Many patients lose their appetite, but some begin to eat compulsively. In either event, weight changes can be significant. Depressed people may sleep excessively, or they may have trouble sleeping. While some can't fall asleep, some others wake repeatedly during the night. Most frequently, patients find themselves awake for the day at four or five in the morning.

When people are depressed, they invariably feel enervated even though they have exerted no physical effort. They may move more slowly than usual and find a task as simple as writing a check too difficult to tackle. Yet, in depression, some people encounter uncontrollable restlessness. They may fidget, pace the floor, wring their hands, pull at their skin or hair. They may burst out shouting, complaining, or expostulating. Conversely, they may become much less verbal than usual, punctuating their infrequent speech with long pauses. Their speech may become slow, droning, monotonal.

The possible profiles of depression are so varied that three depressed people might bear no resemblance to each other. Hal Lear, the urologist whose heart surgery is chronicled in *Heartsounds,* portrays the classic picture of depression, together with the confusing frustration it imposes on family and loved ones. Martha Weinman Lear writes:

> Wearing the same clothes day after day, and surely no accident that they were the dullest-colored things in his

closet. Lying on the bed near-motionless for hours on end, fully dressed, staring at nothing, fiddling mindlessly with the middle button of his shirt, the one over the center of his scar; buttoning and unbuttoning, buttoning and unbuttoning.

I began to grow impatient with him myself. Shave for heaven's sake. Comb your hair. There are worse things in life than a bad memory. . . .

Once I said it aloud. We sat at the table, he poking at his food, and he was trying to say something but the simple word he wanted was not there; he struggled for it and grimaced and banged his head with his fist, crying out, "What has happened to my mind?" and I said, "Oh come on, stop doing that number. It's no tragedy if you can't think of a word."

He looked at me not with anger, which would have been tolerable, but with the deepest sadness. It hurt my eyes. I felt ashamed. . . .

He is going down the tube, and I don't want to go with him [she told a friend]. But I love him. What in God's name do I mean? I didn't understand myself at all.

Like Martha Weinman Lear, who was distraught by her husband's depression, the wife of another patient found herself a helpless bystander during her husband's recovery. Thomas Darling had always felt in charge of his life. After surgery, he felt he had lost control but denied he was depressed. He projected blame for his condition on his wife and made a series of inappropriate, flailing attempts to regain control. As the following letter written by his wife reveals, his depression was hard to recognize.

Within several months of the open-heart surgery, there was a marked change in my husband's personality. Where before he was close with his children and with me, he became distant, not having much to say.  He would take a day off from work and go for a ride alone which is completely out of character.  The family was most patient with him thinking he was just temporarily depressed. . . . He moved out of our home saying he was staying with "friends" (unnamed) because he needed to be alone for a while. . . . Contact with old friends was kept to a minimum and his former great sense of humor was absent. . . . By mid-January he announced that he was marrying a former acquaintance of ours but soon he was again contacting me by phone and we met several times for dinner or a drink. . . . He will now say that he is unhappy and does not know what he wants in life other than to be happy for his few remaining years.  His subsequent physicals have been very good except for a slight extra heartbeat for which he takes medication . . . . He went to the Pritikin Longevity Center in California for two weeks in the hope of finding a correct diet, exercise, and kicking the smoking habit.  He was successful but has gone back to his old habits.  At this point I feel that he definitely does love me and his family, that he is caught up in an affair he wants out of, but I do not know how to help him.

In the cloak of depression, Hilda Tower looks different still.  Although her cardiologist claimed her surgery a success, two months afterwards, she was still having chest pain and some shortness of breath.  Her whole body felt out of synchrony.  Though she was always tired, she could not sleep.  She went to bed at 10:00 only to wake again at 11:00 feeling nervous—so nervous she couldn't stay in bed, so nervous she wanted to bury her head in her pillow and scream.  Although she had been back to work for two weeks, she could not concentrate.

"One day, while I was doing some paperwork, I got nervous for no reason at all," she remembered. "If I hadn't been in an embarrassing situation, I could have cried just as easily as not."

## The Elusiveness of Depression

When the same syndrome can look so different in three people, it's no wonder that health professionals sometimes miss diagnosing it. Yet studies estimate that as many as 32% of all medical patients suffer from serious depression and that up to half of them go unidentified.

The problem is compounded by ambiguity in the term "depression." Since medical professionals sometimes use the word to denote transient sadness, pessimism, or disinterest, the observation that a patient is depressed does not always prompt serious concern. This problem is further confounded when symptoms of depression mirror problems which ordinarily accompany a given medical condition. For example, all patients tire easily after heart surgery. Some report they don't feel like themselves for a year. In addition, bypass patients commonly complain they have no appetite and cannot concentrate. When Albert Peterson complained two months after his operation that he felt listless, his memory was failing, and he couldn't enjoy his favorite foods, was he dangerously depressed or experiencing normal recovery?

Medical professionals sometimes disregard depression because they assume it is consistent with and appropriate to illness, surgery, and recovery. If depression is defined as transient discouragement, this assumption is valid. Certainly, anyone who experiences pain and weakness day after day can have trouble maintaining high spirits. When patients experience setbacks or find their recovery is taking longer than they think it should, they can easily become demoralized. Even someone recovering from the flu can feel discouraged when his knees still wobble two weeks after the fever is gone. But discouragement is not major depression. And while periodic feelings of sadness and demoralization go hand in hand with illness, major depression need not.

Because depression can be so elusive, ambiguous, and

impressionistic, mental health professionals evaluate it by the number and intensity of symptoms which patients exhibit. Generally they refer to the list of nine symptoms in the American Psychiatric Association's *Diagnostic and Statistical Manual* (DSM-III) to determine whether a patient is suffering from this disorder. Professional treatment is indicated when physicians see any five of these symptoms lasting for at least two weeks without relief:

1. A persistent sense of hopelessness and disinterest in stimulating activity;

2. Loss of interest in normally pleasurable activities, apathy, or loss of sex drive;

3. Significant change in appetite patterns, often accompanied by a noticeable change in weight;

4. Change in sleep patterns, either insomnia, disrupted sleep, or sleeping more hours than normal;

5. Apparent nervous energy or muscle sluggishness;

6. Fatigue or lethargy;

7. Feelings of inadequacy or guilt;

8. Difficulty thinking, concentrating, remembering, or making decisions;

9. Preoccupation with death, expressed death wishes, contemplation of or attempts at suicide.

## Depression and Illness

When patients suffer from prolonged debilitating depression, they do not experience the gains their surgery had promised. Several studies affirm that the number of bypass patients who return to work is lower than expected when age, clinical status, and other relevant factors warrant otherwise. Presumably the problem is depression. One study of heart surgery patients with a good physical outcome revealed that 83% were not employed after surgery and 57% were sexually impaired one to two years later. Too many patients who should feel good are significantly limited in their household and leisure activities. They have problems of low self-esteem, prolonged feelings of gloom, and distorted body image—all symptoms of depression.

This phenomenon is not unique to heart surgery. Studies show that one-third of all surgery patients suffer serious debilitating depression. In part, it comes from feelings of helplessness made worse by feelings that privacy has been invaded and dignity stripped away. This is particularly true of people who pride themselves on their independence and their ability to control the events which shape their lives. When these people need to be fed, bathed, and shaved by someone else, the humility can be unbearable. Parenthetically, surgery patients can also experience depression as a side effect of drugs, notably steroids and some heart and high blood pressure medications.

With illness and surgery of the heart, vulnerability to depression is aggravated by the awesome implications of surgery to this vital organ. More than a pump sending life-bearing oxygen throughout the body, it carries mystical significance as the center of the spirit and soul. Consequently, threats to it and tampering with it carry intensified meaning.

People who suffer heart attacks also encounter depression as a significant complication. After the initial threat of death, many worry that their lives have been permanently altered. Some see their illness as a mark of imperfection or confirmation of their inadequacy, and they lose self-esteem. An estimated 60% of patients suffer from anxiety and depression while they are hospitalized; up to 30% remain depressed for a year following their attack. Moreover, some 20% of heart attack patients never return to work, largely because of psychosocial reasons.

Depression and illness form a menacing cycle. Illness causes depression, and in turn, depression can cause heart attacks, according to several studies. For people with angina, the correlation is understandable. This crushing pain, which occurs when oxygen is temporarily diminished in the coronary arteries, serves as a constant warning that the heart is not functioning properly. As the pain comes with exercise, eating, or even during rest, it seems to say, "Be careful. You're vulnerable." Thus people with angina exist in a state of vigilance which can create significant psychological stress.

However, a surprising number of patients with no history of angina are also beset with depression before their heart attacks. Dr. Hal Lear, in *Heartsounds,* was one of them. Trapped in a hopeless work situation, he suddenly burst into tears one day while visiting England. Martha Weinman Lear writes:

> "I hate working for them, I hate them all, I hate the whole damned setup," he had cried, with such an urgent and impotent rage that I should have guessed it might eat like acid into his heart.

The very correlation between depression and heart attacks is one of the factors which prompted our Miami Heart Institute Study.

After surgery, men and women encounter depression at the same rate, although women experience more medical complications than men. However, patients who needed emergency surgery and patients who had no disabling angina before surgery seem to have greater difficulty coping with prolonged recuperation than others. Patients whose lives are littered with problems or who encountered numerous changes over the preceding several months also tend to have a harder time. One patient, for example, was the sole provider for her retarded daughter, who had recently been diagnosed as having a chronic kidney problem and dismissed from the residential school she had attended. In addition, the patient expected to be laid off from her job, and she worried how she would support herself in the future. After surgery, she was depressed to the point of wishing she were dead.

"I worry about my daughter. Who will take care of her and who will take care of me? It would be so easy if I could just close my eyes and not wake up," she cried.

## Overcoming Depression

Patients who overcome their depression easily often attribute their success to good marriages or supportive, perceptive friends. For other patients, the best therapy is going back to work. One patient, who went into his bypass surgery expecting to die and suffered periodic feelings of intense depression for weeks afterwards, believes that going back to work saved his sanity. Many echo this belief. For people who do not work outside the home, putting structure into household work, becoming involved in leisure pursuits, and planning activities with friends offer valuable distractions. Simply breaking the preoccupation with themselves and their bodies often does the trick.

While some depression following surgery is normal and not dangerous, it can become dangerous if it lingers and intensifies. And sometimes, despite monumental efforts to cope effectively, people cannot hold the floodgates of depression secure. The torrent is simply overpowering.

If you lose interest in your favorite activities, take heed. If bad days turn into bad weeks and if these bad weeks are characterized by five of the nine classic symptoms listed earlier in this chapter, you should seek professional help. Turning to a counselor does not imply that you are inadequate or that you have failed in any way. Nor does it suggest that you must spend years in therapy or relinquish control over yourself.

On the contrary, you maintain control because you choose your therapist, who can be a psychologist, psychiatrist, social worker, or member of the clergy. If you are dissatisfied with your choice, you can change. And with the right professional, short-term counseling can be strikingly effective. Likewise, family counseling is often helpful since depression can be as troubling to your family as it is to you. If nothing else, professional intervention permits someone who is not personally involved with you or your family to look at your situation from a new perspective.

To overcome depression, you may need the help of antidepressant drugs for a few months. Again, this is not a sign of bad attitude, ineffective coping, or failure of any other kind. It is a chemical correction to a problem that is largely biochemical in origin. Although antidepressants require the careful supervision of a physician, they are safe drugs that impose few side effects.

Think of antidepressants as keys on a key ring. There are many, and each is somewhat unique. Before you find the right fit, you may have to try several different drugs and a variety of dosages. When you hit upon the right formula, your sleep will improve almost immediately. In about two weeks, you will find yourself noticeably less depressed, and side effects such as dry mouth and constipation will be minimal. Within three to six months, antidepressants can usually reverse the chemical imbalance that perpetuated your depression. The new balance should remain stable after you stop taking the medication.

Whether you shed your depression with or without help, the weights do lift. The tears dry up, the anger fades, and the sun comes out.

## Points to Remember

❑ Reactive depression, much like grief, is usually self-limiting and not dangerous.

❑ In mild cases, social support, returning to work, and becoming involved in other activities are often effective antidotes.

❑ Worrisome depression is measured by the number and duration of its symptoms.

❑ When it is intense, depression forms a menacing cycle with illness and demands professional care.

❑ Brief treatment with antidepressants can cure depression by altering the biochemical balance in the brain.

## Chapter Ten

# PROMOTING RECOVERY AND GOOD HEALTH

It is easy to understand how patients might encounter infection after heart surgery. Likewise, heart arrhythmias, difficulties with blood clots, and a host of other physiological problems seem like logical complications. But depression? Depression is largely emotional. How can emotional difficulty erupt as a complication of physical trauma? If depression is a valid sequel to surgery, there must be an integral connection between the mind and the body.

## Type A Personality

Perhaps the most familiar evidence confirming this connection is the Type A personality. This profile began to emerge in the late 1950s, when California cardiologists Meyer Friedman and Ray Rosenman first observed how quickly the front edges of their waiting room chairs were wearing out. So impatient were their patients, the cardiologists reasoned, that they perched at the edge of their seats ready to pounce forward the moment their names were called.

From this first observation came the now-familiar personality profile. To a large degree, Type A's are the successful men and women in our society. They are ambitious and aggressive, competitive, impatient, and hard-driving. They eat fast and play hard. Frequent interruptions anger them, and they rarely take time to unwind. Instead, they use every minute to get ahead. They make plans while they shower and read while they eat. They hate waiting in line, and when they are in the car, heaven help the driver who slows down in front of them.

The hostility and hard-driving competitiveness characteristic of these people increases their risk of coronary heart disease. So convincing is this correlation that, in 1982, the National Heart, Lung, and Blood Institute issued an official statement about it:

> The review panel accepts the available body of scientific evidence that Type A behavior . . . is associated with increased risk of clinically apparent coronary heart disease in employed, middle-aged, U.S. citizens. The risk is greater than that imposed by age, elevated . . . blood pressure, . . . cholesterol, and smoking, and appears to be in the same order of magnitude as the relative risk associated with the latter of these three factors.

While hostile competitiveness aggravates coronary heart disease, reducing Type A tendencies appears to improve cardiovascular functioning. When Type A business people modified their behavior, they lowered blood pressure and cholesterol levels. Similarly, heart attack victims who learned how to reduce their Type A tendencies suffered fewer subsequent heart attacks than patients who did not.

## The Theory of Stress

These findings are consistent with the first observations correlating stress and physiological changes, which Hans Selye, M.D., Ph.D., made more than half a century ago. In 1926, Hans Selye, the founder and long-time president of the International Institute of Stress, noticed that when laboratory rats were exposed to stress, their adrenal glands enlarged, organs of their immune system shrank, and the animals developed peptic ulcers. Subsequently, experts learned that when people and other animals are in a state of stress, their blood reveals elevated levels of certain hormones, collectively labeled stress hormones, which suppress immunity to illness and endanger various body systems.

How, one might ask, do emotional reactions, which ostensibly take place in the brain, cause changes in hormones, blood, and the functioning of various organs? Truthfully, no one knows for sure. However, numerous studies support a widely accepted theory.

The theory begins with the discovery that thoughts, attitudes, and convictions are correlated with electrochemical events in the brain. Positron emission tomography (PET), which images the metabolism of the brain, can show the brain in action and documents that as mental or cognitive processes change, cerebral blood flow, physiology, and hormonal balance also change. Integral to these electrochemical events are chemical messengers responsible for relaying electrical impulses throughout the nervous system. These messengers are called neurotransmitters.

Neurotransmitters are produced in the brain. They transmit electrical activity within the brain as well as to all other parts of the body. Some of these stimulate glands to secrete hormones, which enter the blood stream and affect all parts of the body, including the immune system, the cardiovascular system, and the brain. Thus, when someone is frightened, neurotransmitters begin a chain reaction which causes him to sweat, his eyes to widen, and his heart rate to increase.

The hormones and neurotransmitters which connect thoughts and emotions to physiological events work as a two-way street. Emotions can trigger an array of physiological occurrences, as the relationship between Type A personality and heart disease illustrates. Conversely, physiological events can alter emotions. When athletes work out, for example, they experience a rush of certain neurotransmitters called endorphins, which are thought to bring on the "runner's high." Because of the resulting sense of well-being, exercise enthusiasts claim that their workouts do as much for their spirits as for their bodies.

In general, it appears that positive emotions promote good health, and vice versa; also that negative emotions promote illness, and vice versa. Moreover, whether emotions are positive or negative depends more on an individual's perception than on an objective analysis of the event which prompted the feelings. Let's look at these factors one at a time.

## Positive Emotions and Good Health

There is increasing evidence that positive emotions strengthen the immune system and thereby promote good health. Harvard psychologist David McClelland discovered that feelings of love and caring increase the body's production of antibodies which fight upper respiratory viruses. Research at the Menninger Clinic suggests that romantic love increases immunity to colds. Romantic love also appears to decrease lactic acid and increase endorphins. These biochemical changes help to explain the vigorous euphoric feelings which often characterize people in love. Faith also seems to promote recovery. A study of patients facing eye surgery revealed that those who expressed trust in their surgeons and their ability to recover healed faster than more skeptical patients. Laughter too has been associated with healing. Since Norman Cousins, renowned author of *Anatomy of an Illness*, first advocated laughter to catalyze recovery, several studies have confirmed the healthy physiological effects of humor. People with good senses of humor exhibit elevated levels of antibodies which protect against colds. Similarly, good moods coincide with the suppression of stress hormones and the elevation of endorphins. So convincing is the therapeutic benefit of laughter that several hospitals have established humor centers. For

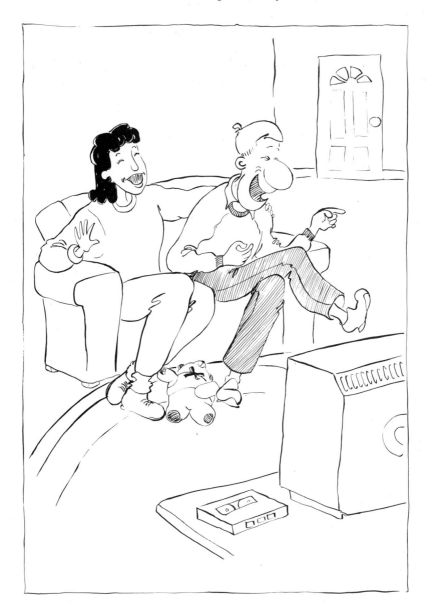

Laughter too has been associated with healing.

example, St Joseph's Hospital in Houston has established the "Living Room" for cancer patients. Equipped with audio and video cassette recorders, the space is a haven for patients to watch comedies and listen to their favorite music.

## Negative Emotions and Illness

Just as feelings of love, optimism, faith, and humor seem to promote well-being, so pervasive feelings of pessimism, anxiety, frustration, conflict, and stress appear to catalyze a variety of illnesses. For example, Harvard Medical School pediatricians observed that among children whose throat cultures tested positive for strep infections, only those who experienced stress were likely to become ill. Similarly, army recruits who developed upper respiratory infections also showed elevated blood levels of stress hormones. And the blood tests of college students who came down with acute infectious diseases revealed a rise in stress hormones before they began to feel sick. Elevated stress hormones are associated with cold sores, migraine headaches, and ulcers. And they can also promote cholesterol buildup and atherosclerosis, a sequence which helps to explain heart disease and Type A personalities.

Perhaps the most potent correlation between negative emotions and ill health is the excessive rate of illness and death among the bereaved. In Australia, the death rate among new widows rose three to twelve times that of their married counterparts. And in England, the death rate for widowers over fifty-four years of age jumped more than 40% in the first six months after the death of their wives. People in grief, like those who suffer from depression, experience weakened immunity to infection as well as a tendency to other physiological difficulties.

These findings coincide with the prevailing theory about how negative emotions alter neurotransmitters and the hormones they affect. Apparently, chronic intense stress, pessimism, and other emotions characteristic of depression affect the brain by depleting the neurotransmitters norepinephrine and dopamine. Moreover, it appears that norepinephrine, dopamine, and a third neurotransmitter, serotonin, play key roles in depression. When optimum amounts of these neurotransmitters fail to travel along the cells in the nervous system, particularly in the front of the brain, the biochemical stage is set for depression. Sleep, appetite, and sex are disrupted. So are moods, movement, motivation, and responsiveness. Even facial expression is altered as depression inhibits control of the muscles around the mouth causing the corners of the mouth to droop.

Several kinds of evidence appear to validate this theory. One, PET scanning reveals that the brain looks different during depression than it does normally. Two mood-elevating drugs commonly used to treat depression, such as Elavil[†] and Tofranil,[‡] work by altering the chemical composition of the brain.

Stress, illness, and depression can form a destructive cycle, but they don't have to. The key to breaking the cycle is perception. When people perceive potential stress as distressing, they increase their vulnerability. If they perceive the potential stress as benign, they do not. Thus, a work load which is overwhelming to one person can seem challenging and stimulating to another. As Harvard University's crisis intervention specialist, Gerald Caplan, observed, when people that feel stress is unmanageable, they begin to feel helpless, and they become vulnerable to depression and illness.

If people can marshal their best coping strategies, they stand the best chance to keep stress in check and thereby prevent the onset of the destructive cycle. This is not to say that people can control the fate of their bodies by improving their attitudes. Attitude, perception, and faith are

[†] Merck Sharp & Dohme (Amitriptyline HCl, MSD USP)
[‡] Geigy (imipramine hydrochloride USP)

only part of a large and complex system including genetics, environment, and other factors over which one has no control. Thus, people who assume full responsibility for their well-being and who imply that, with proper effort, they can achieve immortality, are wrong.

Somewhere between the absurdity that death is optional and the misconception that fate is entirely predestined lies the notion that when people cope effectively, they defuse their distress and enhance their well-being. People can usually reduce their stress when they rely on comfortable coping strategies and adapt these strategies to meet the specific demands of the challenge at hand. Let's take another look at some of the patients we discussed earlier in the book and review ways they adapted their coping styles to manage heart surgery.

## Coping Effectively

Jacques Monteil, the fifty-five-year-old accountant whose experience we quoted from time to time, has an insistent need to intellectualize his stress. By taking an active role in his health care from the moment he first experienced angina, he was able to manage stress without distress. Thus, he began to keep a diary:

> I had always been concerned about my heart, partly because of my family history of heart disease and partly because I have always found the heart particularly intriguing. This thing that moves inside us, without dependence or apparent dependence on our will, is really unique in the human body. And to know that our life depends on the continuity of that movement adds to the awe with which we look upon the heart.

After suffering for years from angina controlled by medication, Jacques Monteil agreed to have an angiogram, again, ostensibly, out of intellectual drive. "My

angina was now at least six years old and . . . one *had* to
know exactly what I had," he wrote in his diary. "No other
means of investigation so far are as accurate and complete
as a film."

Although the angiogram showed several severe blockages, he would not take the recommendation of his cardiologist before he consulted with two others and weighed
their opinions. Once he decided upon surgery and selected
a hospital and surgeon, he set out to prepare for surgery.
He rested, lost weight, and exercised dutifully. He read
*Open Heart Surgery* by Ina Yalof because ". . . the main
source of apprehension and fear is ignorance and surprise,
and this book helped to eliminate both."

After arriving at the hospital, Jacques Monteil met
with his surgeon and made some last-minute preparations for his operation. The entry in his diary reads:

> We had a long talk and he impressed me as knowing my
> file, my history and my angiogram very thoroughly. . . .
> He told me what tests would be done. . . . I knew most of
> this from the book—no surprise.
>
> From my conversations with others who had been oper-
> ated on, I discovered that many could hear the doctors
> speak among themselves in spite of the anesthesia and
> that these conversations later haunted them in their
> dreams. I decided to put cotton wool in my ears to avoid
> this risk. Furthermore, I did not go to sleep too early on
> the day before surgery so as to be still half asleep at the
> time the medication was given to me the day of the
> operation.

By taking such monumental control, Jacques Monteil
set himself up to minimize his distress, and for him it
worked. He recovered with record speed and five years
after his surgery was still healthy, vigorous, and busy
pursuing his career.

In contrast, James Nicholson, whose experiences also appear elsewhere in this text, is much less comfortable assuming responsibility for his care. A mild-mannered, agreeable person who quickly defers to others, he tends to be a quiet worrier. In the stress of impending surgery, he found too much information overwhelming and confusing. He could not find comfort in reading a book on heart surgery or talking to every former patient he encountered. He coped better with small amounts of information repeated often and wrapped in reassurance and encouragement. Thus he filtered out a lot of the information that came his way, and he responded well to comments like, "You'll do just fine." For him, the easiest time was in the ICU; there his natural inclination to dependency was welcomed, and he derived great comfort from the diligent attention of his nurses.

Although everyone has favorite coping strategies, certain strategies are inappropriate in some circumstances. In such instances, the strategy must be modified. For example, since patients come through the earliest postoperative period best when they can depend utterly on their caretakers, patients like Jacques Monteil must modify their instinctive preference for control. These patients often minimize distress by turning their need to control inward. It is patients in this group who are most likely to practice relaxation exercises and self-hypnosis. Since these techniques work best when they have been well practiced, patients whose surgery is elective sometimes practice daily for several weeks. In contrast, people like James Nicholson, who feel comfortable in the dependent role of the ICU patient, often have trouble motivating themselves to take charge of the work inherent in convalescence. These patients can approach advanced recuperation by dutifully obeying orders. When patients effectively adapt their coping strategies to meet the demands of their hospitalization, they come through the experience with a minimum of distress.

Sometimes, people think they are coping well but their behavior belies their perceptions. Such was the case of Paul Stevens, discussed in chapter five. Paul Stevens, who had always been easy-going and reasonable, began having temper tantrums soon after he was moved from the ICU. Though he was not aware he was frightened, his fears were ravaging him. Luckily, his nurse recognized his signals of distress and dealt with them appropriately. When patients persistently behave in a strikingly unusual manner, their ability to cope may be disintegrating and crisis intervention may be helpful.

## Positive Attitude

While coping styles vary among people, certain characteristics appear in all effective coping strategies. Chief among those qualities is a positive attitude. For some, that translates into faith. For others, it's seeing the proverbial glass as half full rather than half empty. For still others, it's choosing to overlook the downside.

"A person at all times has a choice as to what to focus on—foreground or background, good or bad," research psychiatrist Joel Dimsdale observed.

Trying to keep a positive attitude toward surgery helped Michael Strickland, a patient described in chapter three, suppress the fear that sometimes threatened to choke him. "The worst times were at night, when I would lie in bed and feel so panicky. Then I'd just say to myself: Strickland, less than three people in a hundred die from this surgery. You're having the operation because the doctor thinks you're strong enough to do well. You will survive. You will recover. And you will be stronger and healthier than you are now."

Strickland recalled the hypnotic effect the short sentences had on him. You will survive. You will recover, he repeated over and over. Somehow, miraculously, the anxiety subsided for the moment.

Repeating positive statements is a valuable exercise. It can affect the neurochemicals in the brain and begin the chain that promotes well-being. These statements rarely eradicate negative feelings like worry and disbelief. Rather, they offset them and help to put them in perspective.

You can also enhance your sense of well-being by looking at the positive side of your hospitalization, since it is the perception of events, not the events themselves, that creates stress. Hospitalization does have some positive aspects, after all. It may provide a welcome visit from loved ones who live far away. It can be a respite from household chores and an unhurried opportunity to read a good book and listen to some favorite music. Journalist Douglass Cater, who wrote about his surgery in *The New York Times Magazine*, adopted this attitude toward his time in the hospital before surgery. He wrote:

> I have come to treasure the solitude and almost resent the solicitous interruptions of friends and loved ones.... For the first time ever, I have the chance to listen to the same movement [of his favorite Prokofiev, Mozart, and Brahms tapes] over and over again. It has a hypnotic effect, especially during those post-midnight hours when the clock always seems to get stuck.

## Social Support

While social support is invaluable, the kind of support which patients find helpful varies among individuals. Some patients say the best support comes from other patients. Before surgery, they were encouraged when they heard the tales and saw the scars of people who had been to the operating room before them. Fortunately, many former patients find it therapeutic to counsel newcomers to the hospital. Some hospitals also arrange for prospective patients to meet each other in patient education classes and foster communication among them throughout the hospital experience. Peer support groups in cities throughout the country meet this need as well.

While families and close friends offer valuable support to many patients, some, facing severe threats to health, find that support from the people they love most magnifies their sense of incapacity and lowers their self-esteem. These people might do better with support from other patients and health professionals than with sympathetic attention from friends and family. Others need time alone to resolve emotional distress. One patient, for example, dealt with the incessant irritability he felt for months after surgery by going off by himself for a few days. In the mountains, he was able to defuse his anger, and then he returned to his family.

Given the mounting evidence supporting the interaction of the mind and the body, we feel confident that psychological attitudes can affect recovery. The way people cope with surgery does make a difference. Good coping, in one way or another, incorporates sound social support and a positive attitude. When people inject these qualities into their most comfortable coping styles, they enhance their emotional environment and the biochemical foundation which supports it. More than reducing their vulnerability to depression, they boost their recovery from illness and help promote ongoing good health.

## Points to Remember

❑ Thoughts and emotions are products of electrochemical events which connect the mind and the body.

❑ Love, faith, and other positive emotions appear to promote good health while stress and other negative emotions seem to thwart it.

❑ Coping well brings out positive emotions.

❑ Sometimes people must modify their coping strategies to accommodate specific situations.

❑ Constructive coping always incorporates positive attitudes and effective social support.

## Chapter Eleven
# PRESCRIPTION FOR LIFE

Heart surgery has given you new life. Protect it, cherish it, enjoy it.

Under certain circumstances, your heart may be more vulnerable to infection than it used to be. Be sure all your physicians and dentists know about your operation. Before performing treatment as simple as cleaning your teeth, they may want to discuss with your cardiologist the merits of prescribing antibiotics to prevent infection.

If you smoke, *you must find a way to stop.* Admittedly, quitting can be an onerous task. However, there are numerous aids available now. Ask your doctor which are best for you. Your physician may suggest hypnosis and recommend a reputable therapist. Self-help groups, medications which create an aversion to nicotine, and behavior modification are other possibilities. While you may not be able to quit by will-power alone, no method will help you unless you want to quit. Really. Deep down. And if you found the motivation to recover from heart surgery, you ought to be able to find the motivation for this. Please try. Please succeed.

Unfortunately, too many bypass patients make impressive resolutions about reforming their lives in the early months after surgery. As their recovery winds down and the whole unsavory experience fades into history, however, they rationalize their way back into their old, bad habits. This is particularly true of people who regularly resort to denial as a coping mechanism. "Oh, I don't have heart disease. I had my plumbing fixed and now I'm fine," they profess as they devour their eggs benedict. It's a lie, you know. You will always have heart disease. Your arteries will always threaten to shut down and kill you.

Because of the correlation between heart disease and stress, you've got to make a lifetime commitment to hold the lid on tension. Professionals are fond of saying, "Avoid stressful situations." It would be nice if you could, but often you can't. When you feel stress mounting, consciously call on your best coping mechanisms to deal with it. If getting caught in rush hour traffic makes you seethe, get absorbed in the news or a good talk show on the radio. Play a cassette of your favorite music or one of the books on tape that are so readily available these days. Plan your exercise to help diminish stress as well as stimulate your heart. Weave breaks into your business day. Experiment with yoga and relaxation exercises. Attend a stress-management workshop. Investigate behavior modification.

If ever there was an era when maintaining a healthy heart was easy, this is it. As television ads keep reminding us, being fit is in style, and you should find lots of company at the local gym, on the vita course, or walking in your neighborhood before dinner. Increasingly, restaurants are featuring low-cholesterol selections—even omelets made without egg yolks on their brunch menus. McDonald's and Burger King are offering salads. Some ice cream parlors serve delicious cholesterol-free alternatives, and sorbets are in vogue.

Best of all, if you follow an exercise regime and low-fat diet today, you stand a better chance of controlling your cholesterol than ever before. In September 1987, the prescription drug lovastatin became available for general use. After abundant clinical trials, physicians hailed this drug's ability to lower dangerous blood levels of cholesterol when patients also exercise and eat a prudent diet. Moreover, side effects from the drug are minimal. The future looks brighter still. Procter and Gamble is perfecting olestra, a calorie-free, cholesterol-free fat substitute that will taste like fat and cook like fat. Olestra promises to give food all the taste and texture it gets from fat. But instead of putting calories and cholesterol into the body, olestra will actually strip them away. In experimental trials, olestra has reduced blood levels of cholesterol up to 20%.

Other dramatic advances in heart disease management can also help you protect your life. The Cine CT scanner can do one job formerly reserved for cardiac catheterization: It can ascertain whether bypass grafts remain open. If your grafts close, advances in angioplasty may provide non-surgical alternatives to another bypass operation. And in the near future, lasers will literally open a new front in the war on atherosclerosis. Should you have a heart attack, drugs like streptokinase and tissue plasminogen activator (TPA) can often dissolve the clot and prevent damage to the heart muscle. But none of this modern technology and pharmacology can replace your responsibility to yourself.

Stick with your new eating habits. Keep exercising— not just for your heart but for the emotional lift it provides. Dedicate yourself to less stress. Save time for fishing, walking in the woods, visiting grandchildren. If you are retired, become an active volunteer. Read for the blind or tutor some children at a neighborhood school. Take a course at the local college. And for goodness' sake, make time for fun.

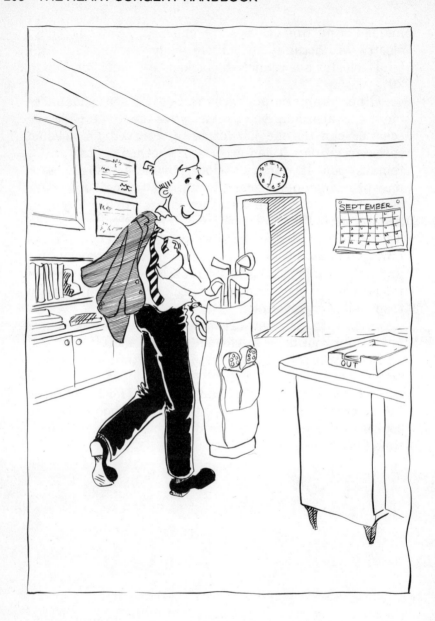

For goodness sake, make time for fun.

# GLOSSARY

**Angiogram:** See cardiac catheterization

**Angina:** Chest pain caused by the temporary constriction of a coronary artery and insufficiency of blood delivered to the heart muscle. Sometimes pain caused by this insufficiency is felt in the left shoulder, left arm, and jaw.

**Anticipatory guidance:** Information provided before an experience which includes details about the events, sensations, and emotions which are likely to occur.

**Anticoagulant:** A drug, such as coumadin or heparin, which retards blood clotting.

**Anti-inflammatory**: Counteracting or suppressing inflammation. Also a drug, such as aspirin or ibuprofen, which counteracts or suppresses the inflammatory process.

**Anxiety**: A pervasive feeling of dread, apprehension, and impending disaster. It can cause muscles to become tense, breathing faster, and the heart to beat more rapidly.

**Aorta**: The main trunk of the artery system. The aorta sends freshly oxygenated blood from the heart to the lesser arteries, which in turn deliver it throughout the body. When vein grafts are used for bypass, one end of each graft is connected to the aorta. The other end is connected to the occluded coronary artery below the point of blockage.

**Arrhythmia**: An irregular or abnormal heartbeat.

**Artery**: A blood vessel which carries blood from the heart to another part of the body.

**Ascending aorta**: The part of the aorta closest to the left ventricle. This vessel, which handles blood rich with fresh oxygen, feeds the coronary arteries.

**Atherosclerosis**: The condition in which plaque builds up within the arteries. As a result of atherosclerosis, arteries harden and narrow. The resulting disease is also called arteriosclerosis or hardening of the arteries.

**Autoimmune response**: The phenomenon by which the body's immune system attacks its own tissues. This sometimes occurs as a reaction to surgery, is responsible for postcardiotomy syndrome, and is reversible with medication. (See postcardiotomy syndrome below.)

**Cardiac catheterization**: The procedure by which a thin tube is threaded through a major artery and vein (usually in the leg but sometimes in the arm) to the heart for the purpose of introducing a radio-opaque dye, which permits an x-ray of the heart and arteries that feed it. This film reveals the circulation of the heart as well as blockages and clues about the efficiency of the heart muscle's pumping capabilities.

**Carotid arteries**: The major arteries which feed the head and brain.

**Cholesterol**: A fatty substance that is essential to the structure and functioning of the human body. Cholesterol is manufactured in the liver and transported elsewhere in the body by two carriers: high-density lipoproteins (HDL) and low-density lipoproteins (LDL). LDLs carry cholesterol from the liver and deposit it throughout the body. Too many LDLs result in excessive cholesterol buildup in the body, especially inside the arteries, setting the stage for atherosclerosis. HDLs, in contrast, carry cholesterol from throughout the body back to the liver, enabling the body to eliminate it. Abundant HDLs reduce the risk of atherosclerosis. The lower your cholesterol count and the proportion of LDLs, the lower your risk of cholesterol contributing to heart disease.

**Circulation**: The process by which blood carries oxygen and other fuels to cells throughout the body and picks up carbon dioxide and other waste products for disposal. Circulation centers in the heart and lungs. Freshly oxygenated blood flows from the lungs through the pulmonary veins, into the upper left chamber of the heart, or left atrium, and then down into the all-important left ventricle. This powerful chamber pumps the blood into the aorta and from there throughout the body. On its return trip, blood laden with carbon dioxide returns to the heart through the vena cava, or main vein. It is collected in the upper right chamber of the heart, or right atrium. From there, it travels into the lower right chamber, the right ventricle, and then, via the pulmonary artery, into the lungs. In the lungs, carbon dioxide is exchanged for oxygen and the process begins anew.

**Congestive heart failure**: A condition characterized by the inability of the heart to pump blood effectively to the body's tissues. Congestive heart failure causes decreased production of urine and retention of fluid in the lungs, abdomen, and legs. The condition is treated with digitalis to improve the heart's pumping capacity and diuretics to rid the body of excess fluid. Symptoms of congestive heart failure sometimes occur after heart surgery because of the surplus of fluids pumped into the body during the operation.

**Coping**: The schemes and strategies people may employ in response to stress. While coping, in the vernacular, implies success, the denotation of the term does not. Thus, breaking down a large problem into manageable components is a coping strategy, and often a successful one. But, technically speaking, smoking and nail biting are coping strategies as well.

**Coronary**: Also called a heart attack or myocardial infarction. It refers to the occlusion of a coronary artery from a blood clot or atherosclerotic debris and results in damage to part of the heart muscle. Recent medical advances can reduce muscle damage if treatment is instituted immediately.

**Coronary arteries**: The first branches off the ascending aorta, which feed fresh blood to the muscle of the heart. Confusion about circulation often occurs because the heart pumps blood throughout the body but also needs blood for its own nourishment. The heart, after all, is a muscular organ and, like any organ, needs its own healthy circulation to flourish. This circulation is managed by the two coronary arteries and their branches. The right coronary artery and its subsidiaries feed the right atrium and the right ventricle, which sends blood to the lungs to be replenished with oxygen. The all-important left main artery feeds the powerful left side of the heart. The left atrium, which receives oxygenated blood from the lungs, is fed by some branches of the left circumflex artery. Because the pumping capability of the left ventricle is integral to the efficiency with which the blood is delivered throughout the body, unobstructed blood flow through the left main coronary artery and its primary branches is particularly important.

**Crisis**: A situation or event that produces stress. During crisis, people stop functioning in their usual ways. They become overwhelmed and feel anxious. They have trouble solving problems and setting priorities, and, as a result, feel helpless.

**Crisis intervention**: Short-term counseling specially designed to help people solve the problems which seem insurmountable in the context of crisis. This therapy incorporates anticipatory guidance, problem solving, conceptual information, and the encouragement of social support. Although crises usually aggravate other existing problems, crisis intervention does not deal with those problems. Its goal is to return the person in crisis to his or her precrisis state.

**Denial**: The conscious or unconscious refusal to accept the existence of anxiety-producing events, ideas, or feelings.

**Depression**: A psychological state often characterized by some combination of the following: dejected mood, disinterest in normally stimulating activities, sleep and appetite disturbances, low energy, difficulties thinking and concentrating, feelings of inadequacy and guilt, and medical complaints.

**Diuretic**: A drug, such as Lasix,* which rids the body of excess fluid and sodium.

**Edema**: Swelling caused by excessive fluid in the body.

**Electrocardiogram (EKG)**: A graphic representation of the electric current produced by the heart.

**Electrolytes**: Chemicals including sodium, potassium, chloride, bicarbonate, calcium, and magnesium which exist in a dissolved state in the blood and other body fluids. In order for the body to function properly and for a person to feel well, electrolytes must be properly balanced. Surgery may prompt a temporary imbalance, which can trigger an array of uncomfortable but correctable symptoms.

**Femoral artery**: One of the main arteries of the leg located near the groin. This is the artery usually entered for cardiac catheterization, though the brachial artery, located on the inner side of the arm, is sometimes used.

**Fibrillation**: Erratic electrical activity of the heart in which inefficient contracting of the heart muscle diminishes the heart's ability to pump.

**Heart-lung machine**: The mechanical device which exchanges carbon dioxide for oxygen in the blood and pumps reoxygenated blood through the body while the heart is stopped during surgery.

**Intubate**: To insert a tube between the vocal cords and into the windpipe. The other end of this tube is connected to a respirator, which controls breathing for patients during surgery and for several hours afterwards.

* Hoechst-Roussel (furosemide)

**Left main coronary artery**: The source of fresh blood to the entire left side of the heart. (See definition for coronary arteries above.) Blockage of this artery is a dire threat to life.

**Left ventricle**: The very muscular chamber of the heart which pumps freshly oxygenated blood throughout the body. (See definition for circulation above.)

**Mammary arteries**: The two arteries running alongside the breast plate (sternum). They feed the chest wall and are sometimes used for bypass grafts. The mammary artery takes longer to prepare for use as a graft but it is likely to remain unclogged for a greater number of years than the saphenous vein, the other vessel commonly used for bypass.

**Neurological difficulties**: Any of numerous problems emanating from the brain possibly associated with heart surgery. These range from stroke to transient difficulties concentrating and include numbness, tingling, and weakness in the limbs; speech difficulties; and slowed thinking, confusion, and memory loss. These problems are rarely severe and seldom permanent.

**Nitroglycerine**: A drug commonly used to treat angina. It is administered by tablet, which is placed under the tongue; long-acting capsule, which is swallowed; or transdermal patch, worn like a Band-Aid on the skin. Nitroglycerine dilates the arteries temporarily, thus improving blood flow to the heart and relieving chest pain.

**Nuclear scan**: A variety of x-ray studies incorporating radioisotopes, which are injected into the blood stream, to reveal the functioning of the heart. These tests can accurately measure the efficiency of the heart pump and show areas where the muscle has been injured. While nuclear scans often fit into a thorough diagnostic work-up, they cannot take the place of cardiac catheterization because only catheterization can reveal blockages in the coronary arteries.

**Oxygenation**: The process of infusing blood with oxygen, which takes place in the lungs.

**Pacemaker**: An electrical device used to maintain the electric impulse when the heart cannot do so independently. Two thin wires affixed to the heart temporarily during surgery are connected to an external pacemaker, which is often needed to regulate the heartbeat for several days after surgery. When the electrical system of the heart proves to be permanently unreliable, a tiny internal pacemaker can be surgically implanted near the heart.

**Palpitations**: See arrhythmia.

**Paranoia**: The presence of delusions. Patients occasionally experience paranoia in the ICU. This is a transient problem experienced most commonly by the elderly and caused, in part, by poor circulation in the brain as a result of enforced bed rest. Once patients are moved to a regular hospital room and spend some time out of bed, these delusions almost always disappear.

**Platelet**: A type of blood cell critical to blood clotting.

**Pleurisy**: An inflammation of the membrane which lines the chest cavity accompanied by fluid exuded into the cavity. The condition can occur as a complication of heart surgery and is characterized by pain in the side, a chill, fever, dry cough. As the condition worsens, pain lessens, but, as fluids build up, breathing becomes difficult.

**Postcardiotomy syndrome**: A common complication which can set in during the first weeks after surgery. It is characterized by fever and other flu-like symptoms. Chest pain and depression may also occur.

**Projection**:  A mental mechanism by which people repress emotions or attitudes into their subconscious and view them as coming from someone else.

**Psychosis**:  A severe mental disorder.  After bypass surgery, patients occasionally experience psychosis briefly in the form of paranoia (See above).

**Right atrium**:  The chamber of the heart which receives blood laden with waste products. (See circulation above.) While the heart-lung machine is in operation, blood is routed into the machine via a tube inserted into an opening in this chamber.

**Saphenous vein**:  A large, superficial, non-essential vein in the leg which is often used for coronary artery grafts in bypass surgery.  There are two saphenous veins in each leg.  One runs from the thigh to the foot and the other from the knee to the foot.

**Stress test**:  Assessment of the capability of the heart to withstand exercise.  The patient confronts increasingly challenging exercises while an electrocardiogram traces the electrical activity of the heart.  Sometimes a nuclear scan is coordinated with this study.

**Subclavian vein**:  The large vein at the base of the neck.  In preparation for heart surgery, a catheter is threaded through this vein, into the heart, and then into the pulmonary artery to assess how the heart is functioning during the operation.

**Vein**:  A vessel which carries blood from other parts of the body to the heart.

# APPENDIX II
# DIAGRAMS

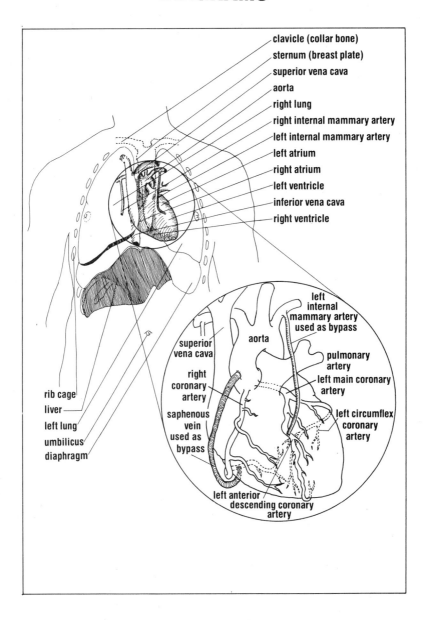

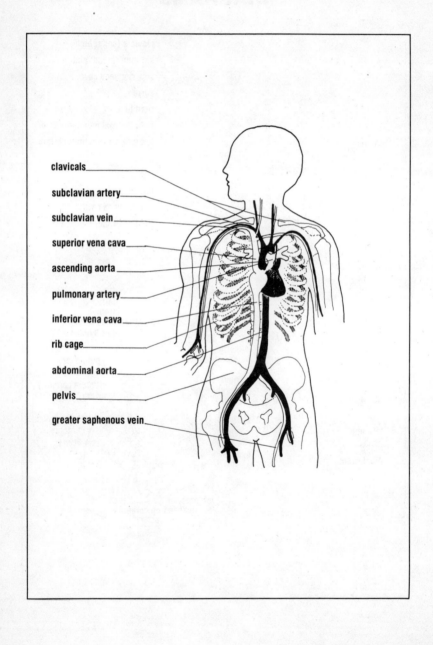

clavicals

subclavian artery

subclavian vein

superior vena cava

ascending aorta

pulmonary artery

inferior vena cava

rib cage

abdominal aorta

pelvis

greater saphenous vein

APPENDIX III
# SOME ADDITIONAL RESOURCES

Benson, Herbert, M.D., and Miriam Z. Klipper. *The Relaxation Response* New York: Avon Books, 1975. The theory and practice of one approach to relaxation.

Blacher, Richard S. *The Psychological Experience of Surgery*. New York: John Wiley and Sons, 1987. An in-depth discussion designed for medical professionals, but nonetheless meaningful to lay readers.

Brody, Jane. *Jane Brody's Nutrition Book* and *Jane Brody's Good Food Book: Living the High Carbohydrate Way*. New York: Bantam, 1987. The most recent information on nutrition with sound tips for converting to a more healthful eating style.

*Cardiac Alert*. Jorge C. Rias, M.D., Ed. (Phillips Publishing, Inc., 7811 Montrose Road, Potomac, MD) Published monthly to provide timely, accurate information about heart disease prevention, diagnosis, and treatment.

Claiborne, Craig with Pierre Franey. *Craig Claiborne's Gourmet Diet*. New York: Times Books, 1980. Two hundred specially created low-sodium, modified-fat, modified cholesterol recipes, each with an analysis of cholesterol, fat, sodium, and calorie content.

DeBakey, Michael, et al. *The Living Heart Diet*. New York: Simon and Schuster, 1977. A complete discussion of the correlation between diet and health plus hundreds of recipes divided among several diet plans each of which is specifically geared for lowering calories, lowering salt, lowering sugar, or sharply reducing fats.

Fensterheim, H., and J. Baer. *Stop Running Scared*. New York: Dell Publishing Company, Inc., 1978. Although this book addresses mental health problems, it offers excellent self-help materials for managing anxiety and fear; these materials are applicable to the heart surgery experience.

Halperin Jonathan L., M.D., and Richard Levine. *Bypass*. Tucson: The Body Press, 1985. A comprehensive, intellectual discussion of heart disease and heart surgery. The discussion of some of the difficulties of recovery and returning to work is especially good.

*Harvard Medical School Health Letter*. William I. Bennett, M.D., Ed. (Department of Continuing Education, Harvard Medical School, Boston, MA) Published monthly to disseminate and interpret medical news.

*Health Letter*. Sidney Wolf, Ed. (The Health Research Group, Washington, D.C.) Published monthly to help consumers make knowledgeable decisions about their health.

Hoffman, Nancy Yanes. *Change of Heart: The Bypass Experience*. New York: Harper and Row, 1985. Twenty-one case histories of bypass patients plus imaginative tips for handling some aspects of the experience.

Justice, Blair. *Who Gets Sick: Thinking and Health*. Houston: The Peak Press, 1987. A narrative discussion of the mind-body connection with summary references to numerous studies.

Long, James W., M.D. *The Essential Guide to Prescriptions*. New York: Harper and Row, 1987. An encyclopedic guide written specifically for lay people. It includes a comprehensible discussion of uses, doses, dosage instructions, contraindications, side effects, adverse reactions, and more.

Nora, James J., M.D., M.P.H. *The Whole Heart Book*. New York: Holt, Rinehart and Winston, 1980. A comprehensive guide to healthful living, including diet, smoking, blood pressure, stress control, and exercise.

Pimm, June B., and Joseph R. Feist. *Psychological Risks of Coronary Bypass Surgery*. New York: Plenum, 1984. A thorough presentation of the Miami Heart Institute Study.

Sunshine, Linda, and John W. Wright. *The Best Hospitals in America*. New York: Henry Holt and Co., 1987. A discussion of what makes a hospital great and an annotated listing of sixty-four outstanding medical institutions.

*The Tufts University Diet and Nutrition Letter*. Stanley N. Gershoff, Ph.D., Ed. (Tufts University School of Nutrition, Medford, MA) Published monthly to disseminate the latest findings on diet and nutrition.

Yalof, Ina L. *Open Heart Surgery*. New York: Random House, 1983. Includes easy-to-understand descriptions of the various diagnostic tests relevant to heart disease and complications which can follow surgery. Also a comprehensive list of resources.

# INDEX

Insomnia 17, 108, 138-39,
146, 152, 178, 181, 183, 185
Intensive Care Unit (ICU) 13,
14, 67-82, 83, 85, 90, 94, 95,
98, 106, 148, 156, 160-63,
174, 200, 201
Items to bring to 161-162
Intubation (see also Endotracheal tube) 40-41, 68-73,
161-62, 213

Kolitz, Sally 13-14, 94, 154,
173

Lear, Martha Weinman 73,
79, 143, 181-82, 187

Mammary artery 31, 66, 214
Medications 26-27, 30, 31-33,
75, 77, 87, 96, 87, 103, 111,
136-37, 146, 186, 198
antidepressant 189-90,
197
pain 5, 46, 73, 86, 87, 88,
95, 100, 124
sleep 139
Memory loss 79, 95, 96, 97,
103, 111, 118, 119, 184, 185
Mended Hearts 147, 150
Miami Heart Institute Study
1-4, 6, 8, 12-17, 114, 187
Monteil, Jacques 28, 30-31,
198-99, 200
Muscle strain 96, 115
Myocardial infarction (see
Heart attack)

Naso-gastric tube 65, 160-61
Neurotransmitters 193-94,
196-97
Nicholson, James 88, 200
Nitroglycerine 32, 89, 169,
214
Numbness in the chest 96,
105, 115

Oxygen 66, 70, 72, 81

Pacemaker 67, 215
Pain (see also Discomfort) 8,
23, 26, 27, 68, 86, 87, 88, 89,
90, 96, 100, 105, 108, 109,
115, 124, 167, 184
Panic 70, 178, 179
Paranoia 76-77, 215
Patient education 5-6, 46-47,
52, 61, 103, 155, 156, 203
Personality 13, 31-33
change 15, 59, 93, 170,
171
Positive attitude 32, 116-17,
201-02, 203, 204
statements to reinforce 49-
50, 62, 70, 202
*Psychological Risks of Coro-
nary Bypass Surgery* 4
Psychological tests 3, 12-13
Psychosis 76-98
Pulmonary artery 211-216
Pulmonary vein 211
Pulse, taking and rcording
127

Razin, Andrew 59

Reading, difficulty with 95
*Recent Life Changes*
  *Questionnaire* 3
Recovery, responsibility for
  171-72
Regression 109
Resentment 169-171, 172
Respiration 31, 68
Respirator 65, 68-73
Rest 75, 86, 104, 106, 108-
  109, 119, 123-129, 131, 137,
  145, 150, 152, 161, 171
Retirement 93, 117, 148
Rib cage 65, 96, 115
Right atrium 65, 66, 216
Right ventricle 211, 212
*Rotter Locus of Control Scale*
  3

Saphenous vein 31, 66, 216
Second opinion 30-32, 69,
  147-47, 199
Sedation 22, 61, 63
Self-control (see also Control)
  14, 15, 53, 81, 93, 95, 96,
  109
Self-esteem 10, 45, 186, 187,
  203
Setbacks (see also Complications) 79, 90, 93, 93, 100,
  104, 114, 154, 165, 184,
Sex 90, 114, 128, 142-146,
  152, 185, 186, 197
Sitting up, technique for 47-
  49, 61
Sleep (see also Insomnia) 75,
  123-24, 181, 185, 189, 197

Smoking 21, 97-98, 192, 205
Social support (see also
  Emotional support) 154-55,
  190, 202-04, 212
Splinting the incision 47, 61,
  73
Stairs, climbing 128, 145
Stevens, Paul 90-91, 93, 201
Stress 4, 13, 14, 15, 21, 50,
  52, 83, 95, 96, 100, 103, 109,
  111, 116, 146, 150, 151, 153-
  54, 156, 165, 167, 173-74,
  177, 192-98, 200, 201, 203,
  206, 211, 212
  hormones 193, 194, 196-98
  test 21, 22, 32, 216
Strickland, Michael 55, 56,
  201
Stroke 25, 32, 78-79
Subclavian vein 64, 216
Support groups 18, 116, 129,
  146-147, 152, 203

Telemetry 85, 98
Type A personality 191-192,
  196

Vena cava 211

Weakness 88, 90, 95, 96, 100,
  105, 108, 114, 159, 184
Work, discrimination at 150-
  152
Work, return to 90, 117, 129,
  148-152, 167, 187, 190

Yalof, Ina 28, 199

# AUTHORS' NOTE

Because the study which inspired this book was restricted to bypass patients, much of this book is devoted specifically to this type of surgery. However, most of the experiences and reactions pertain to all heart surgery patients, and, to a great extent, all surgery patients. In fact, several patients quoted in this book underwent valve replacement or the repair of heart defects, not bypass per se. Except for people whose experiences have previously been published, patients' names and other identifying features have been changed to protect their privacy.

Carol Cohan, M.A., first became involved with the Miami Heart Institute Study as a medical writer in 1984. James Jude M.D. served as medical consultant during the original research and as a guiding spirit for this book. June Pimm Ph.D., together with Joseph Feist Ph.D., designed and led the study. Thus, the first person is used with editorial license.